Homeopathy - Nature's Way to Better Health

Vol. 1

Editing by Saacha Belgar
and Jeannette Susor

Layout and design by
DEVIN RICE DESIGNS

Cover photo - statue of Samuel Hahnemann in Washington D.C.
1755-1843

Purpose

The purpose of this book is to give easy access to the knowledge of the most common first aid homeopathic medicines.

DEDICATION

To my teachers and all those who helped
in this project.

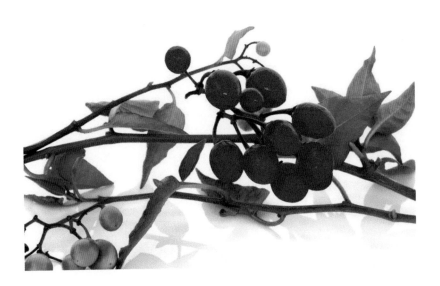

TABLE OF CONTENTS

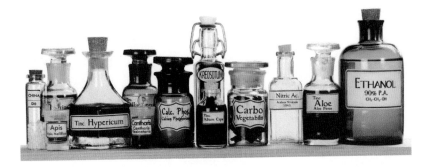

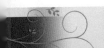

PREFACE

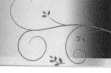

This book is a starting point for those who would like to learn how to use homeopathic medicines to treat common first aid ailments such as pain from injuries, burns, food poisoning, nausea, wounds etc.

For minor ailments these remedies can greatly speed up the healing process, relieve pain and prevent complications. In some more severe cases the correct remedy will reduce pain so that addictive pain drugs can be avoided. Here are two examples:

In one case I treated a patient who had put his palm on a hot muffler. The skin was blistered and he had to hold onto ice to alleviate some of the pain. The *Cantharis 30c* helped for about a minute each time it was taken. The 200c worked for a bit longer but after *Cantharis 1M* the pain was permanently reduced by 95%. He did not need to take any other pain medication or even have to take the *Cantharis 1M* again. I have used this remedy successfully many times for burn pain and now you can too.

Sports injuries are very common. I once was running in a park and was turned backward to catch a Frisbee. Then I ran into a concrete park bench. The pain where my leg hit the bench was severe. I also felt pain all through my body. After *Arnica 200c,* the pain was 90% relieved in about a minute. The next day there was no bruising on that leg! This is a typical story for *Arnica*. It is the most popular remedy because physical trauma is so common.

I have used every remedy in this book I many times. They have all been used in this manner by homeopathic doctors over the past 200 years for the same conditions with great success.

Homeopathy is based on the idea that the body can heal itself. One could say the body usually does heal itself, but when it can't (because of trauma or stress) then it is best to find something that will stimulate the healing system to regain all of its abilities.

This is a very simple idea:

All healing is self-healing.

In fact, the body does regulate itself. In science this is called homeostasis. There is something very fundamental, satisfying and permanently good when one can make homeostasis stronger and intelligent again, so that self-healing can resume and go along its merry way.[1]

"I feel better. My vitality is restored, my symptoms have abated and I am in a positive state of mind again."

Over the past 200 years this is what patients around the world have claimed when they receive the correct homeopathic medicine. Over 25 years as a practitioner, I have seen this happen hundreds of times a year. It is quite thrilling especially if the illness they had was chronic and severe.

"Thank you for helping me – You have no idea how much you have changed my life!"

Patients often ask me how it works and how can one learn this method to treat fist aid and acute ailments?

It is a very powerful and a well thought out approach. When a person is sick many of the body's resources are searching for that one key or bit of information to allow the healing system to complete the self-cure.

The healing system is intelligent – if you give it exactly the right thing – a specific key- something amazing will happen!

In 1790 Samuel Hahnemann discovered how to find this exact

---

1   In chronic ailments this is even more crucial as the correct remedy or remedies will mean the ailment is not passed onto the next generation.

key and how to prepare a medicine so that it could work with the body to jump start the healing process. This is what he found out: when a person is sick it is best to give them a small dose of the same substance that could make them get exactly the same symptoms or sickness – but give it in an extremely small dose.

> Give the patient the similar medicine – it
> will cure them.

He called this the

> Law of healing or Law of Cure.

That being:

> Likes are cured with likes.

Or in Latin:

> Similia Similibus Curentur

The name of this medicine is called:

> The simillimum or most
> similar remedy

Let me give you some examples:
- If cutting onions can make the eyes burn, then a small dose of this same substance will cure the burning eyes of hay fever.
- If Ipecac can cause nausea, then a small dose can cure nausea.
- If coffee can wake you up, then in a small dose it can cure people who feel too awake. In other words, help someone to fall asleep.[2]

How is this possible? Consider an athlete. If we asked a person who had never trained to run a marathon or 26 miles, they most

---

2   Actually the totality of the symptoms of the patient have to fit the total symptoms of the medicine – not just one symptom.

likely could not do it. They may injure themselves, or at the very least, would feel overwhelmed by such a task. The muscles, the following day, would be sore. They may have a sprain, weakness or even strained the heart. If we took the same person and put them on an incremental training program for over a year – a small dose – they could very easily complete a marathon and not suffer any negative effects.

Small doses stimulate and are of benefit
while large doses are toxic.

This is true for any substance and any type of stress. Edward Calabrese who studies the phenomenon of hormesis calls this a:

Universal principle.

Therefore, in homeopathy, we find that the small dose, minimum dose or infinitesimal dose, is what works best.

Large doses or a large stress will produce symptoms while a small dose can make you stronger.

Think again of the runner. A small dose of exercise every day leads to building up and stronger capacity in the muscles, lungs and heart.

How can this help us with diseases or injuries?

If we could find a medicine and use it in a small dose for every part of the healing system we could treat any disease.

Normally we think of identifying a condition such as cancer, and then try to find a cure for it. This is backwards thinking. It will never work for cancer. It will never work for a sprained ankle, ear ache, or for any other illness.

It is better to find out what each medicine will cure
and then apply it to the person who needs it.

What each medicine will cure is never going to change. What is variable is each patient. How can we determine what each medicine will cure?

Nature provides so many plants, minerals and other sources of medicines.

Any substance can be made into a homeopathic medicine, such as silica, sulfur, gold, silver, iron, sodium or plants such as Wind Flower, Rosemary and Club Moss. So far, we have studies of over 3,000 individual medicines. About twelve of them are amazingly effective for first aid. Many more are for colds, flu and various other infections and chronic ailments.

How do we find out what each medicine will cure?

In 1790, Hahnemann was interested in finding out why quinine (derived from the bark of a tree) was effective in treating malaria. He took some and developed some symptoms of malaria.

"I took, by way of experiment, twice a day, four drams[3] of good China (Cinchona). My feet, finger ends, etc., at first, became cold; I grew languid and drowsy, then my heart began to palpitate, and my pulse grew hard and small; intolerable anxiety, trembling, prostration, throughout all my limbs; then pulsation in the head, redness of my cheeks, thirst, and in short, all these symptoms which are ordinarily characteristic of intermittent fever, made their appearance, one after the other, yet without the peculiar chilly, shivering rigor, briefly, even those symptoms which are of regular occurrence and especially characteristic - as the dullness of mind, the kind of rigidity in all the limbs, but above all the numb, disagreeable

---

3   Hahnemann took four drams of Cinchona in 1790. This represents fifteen grams of Peruvian bark in crude form. The pharmaceutical in 1790 was powdered bark of mostly Cinchona officinalis with about 3% of quinine content. This means approximately 0.4 grams of quinine, which is equivalent to a single therapeutic dose. If 100% equals 14.904 grams, then 3% represents 0.447 grams. Http://www.angelfire.com/mb2/quinine/allergy.html

sensation, which seems to have its seed in the periosteum, over every bone in the body - all these made their appearance. This paroxysm lasted two or three hours each time, and recurred if I repeated this dose, not otherwise. I discontinued it, and was in good health."

Hahnemann concluded:

If Quinine can create malaria-like symptoms in a healthy person then it can cure those same symptoms in a sick person.

Quinine happens to be that substance that makes the healing systems of the body or homeostasis stronger against an illness like malaria. If each medicine is studied with the same method; by giving it in large doses to healthy people, then we can determine what it will cause, and in so doing, find out what it will cure in a very low dose.

Since this first study with quinine in1790, we have found out through this same method of 'provings' all about the thousands of medicines we use. Diluted remedies are used to find out what symptoms they can temporarily cause. The variation of symptoms produced, one can imagine, is astonishing because:

There are so many different medicines, therefore, this tells us that there are so many different ways in which the healing system can be broken and healed.

In some remedies the effects are mostly physical. We found out that *Calendula officinalis* cures the effect of cuts and scrapes, prevents infections of those types of injuries and even takes away most of the pain after surgery. Other remedies, such as *Ignatia amara,* affect mostly the emotions. This remedy is one of the best for the sudden shock of grief when the person can't eat or sleep from sadness; they often have a lump in the throat and the moods are very changeable. Other remedies are of benefit to the mind to help memory or help one concentrate.

What follows is a list of the common conditions and each remedy, which time and again, have helped the healing systems of the body recover from those ailments. After using them all a few times, you most likely will not have to look them up. They become old friends that don't change.

You will soon find out that the same remedy can be used in many different situations because the remedy does not treat the symptoms. It only makes the healing system stronger. When it is stronger the body cured itself.

ADVANTAGES TO USING HOMEOPATHY

EASY TO TAKE
Homeopathic medicines are given either as small pleasant tasting tablets which dissolve in the mouth, or in liquid form. Granules or drops are available for babies and children.

INEXPENSIVE
Homeopathic medicines cost surprisingly less than allopathic prescription medication.

NOT TESTED ON ANIMALS
Humans and animals respond differently to medications. All homeopathic medication are tested on healthy humans.

THE MEDICINE OF THE FUTURE
Homeopathy is a growing science and art. There are over 3,000 homeopathic medicines in existence. New homeopathic medicines are being discovered all the time. However, unlike allopathic medicine that take drugs off the market every year as new side-effects are discovered, homeopaths still use the same medicines they were using 200 years ago with new medicines to broaden their scope.

FAMOUS PEOPLE WHO HAVE USED HOMEOPATHY
The Royal Family of Great Britain, Mahatma Gandhi, Mother

Theresa, Mark Twain, Tina Turner, John D. Rockefeller Sr and Paul McCartney just to name a few.

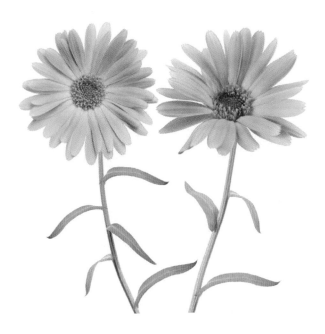

Calendula Officinalis

CHAPTER 1

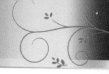

The Practice of Homeopathy for First Aid Conditions

THE THREE PRINCIPLES OF HOMEOPATHY

1. The Single Remedy. It is best to only use one medicine at a time. If two are used at the same time, then the effect may be partial, one may antidote the other. If we want to use a stronger version of one of them there is no way to know which one to make stronger.

2. The Minimum Dose. As the body is already reacting to the illness before any medicine is taken (it has already decided how it wants to get better), it only needs a small dose to make this healing reaction stronger and only the minimum number of doses taken. As we shall see a 30c is a small dose. It is useful for almost all the ailments discussed in this book. Usually only one dose is needed and only repeated if the symptoms return, or the healing reaction stops before all the symptoms are better.

3. The Similar Remedy. The remedy has to match nearly all of the patients unique and unusual symptoms. For example, Arnica montana treats pain that results from a sprain with 'bruised soreness' worse from touch and worse from cold. Ledum pulustre also treats pain from injuries with bruising but better from cold applications. The more unique characteristics one can learn about each remedy the easier it is to know when it is needed.

WHO USES HOMEOPATHY?

Anyone can use homeopathy – babies, pregnant women, the elderly.

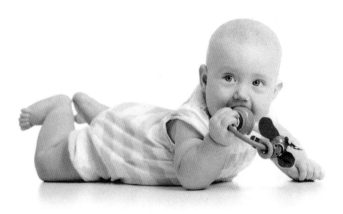

WHEN TO SELF-TREAT? WHEN TO GET A PROFESSIONAL OPINION?

Every case requires its own evaluation. Take the remedy which is indicated and wait to see if there is some improvement within a reasonable amount of time. For a first aid situation, this should happen within a couple of hours. With an acute condition, such as a cold or ear infection, this should happen within 24 hours – usually by the following morning. If any medical condition is deteriorating, or shows signs of worsening, then seek out a licensed naturopath, homeopath, chiropractor or other health professional. In some situations, it may be better to call 911 first and then give the most indicated remedy.

HOW TO DIAGNOSE A FIRST AID CASE

The most important thing to find out is;

What happened –

What is the story behind the ailment? Most of the time this story alone will indicate what remedy is needed. It is enough to identify how the injury or illness occurred? Was it physical trauma, over-exposure to sun, nausea after eating, surgery pain? Each remedy has a story and this can be used to match up with the story of how the ailment came about.

Example: Your nine year old daughter was playing soccer. She tripped, fell on her shoulder and bumped her head. First remedy to give is Arnica 30c as this is the first remedy to give after any physical trauma.

The second thing to find out is:

WHICH TISSUES ARE PRIMARILY INVOLVED?

Find out what tissue is damaged.

Each first aid remedy mostly treats a specific tissue. Arnica: muscles and joints. Hypericum: nerves. Ruta: connective tissue. Symphytum: bone, tendons and ligaments. Calendula: skin.

WHAT ARE THE MAIN SYMPTOMS?

Pain? Stiffness? Weakness? Swelling? Make a list of these main symptoms.

What affects each symptom.

What makes each symptom better or worse? Such as, is the pain worse or better from motion? Worse or better from cold and heat? Each remedy usually has a few of these worse or better from symptoms. We call these modalities. For example Bryonia is always worse from motion, even a very small motion such as walking with a sprained ankle.

How to make an analysis of the symptoms

Look at the totality of the symptoms, both physical and emotional. For example, look for what is unusual about the symptoms.

When there is a fever look for hot head, cold hands (Belladonna). Look for what is intense and clear about the symptoms. Finally, choose one remedy and give it. If you took or gave the correct one, you will see or feel a lot of positive changes in a short amount of time. If you took or gave the incorrect one, it can't do any harm. If it does not help at all after 12 to 24 hours, then give a different remedy. The more severe the situation, the quicker the remedy should act. For example, if someone is in shock and having a panic attack after a car accident, then the remedy - usually Aconite - should help in a matter of ten minutes or so.

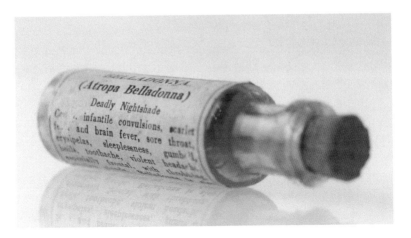

Medicines – homeopathic - how are they made?

A 'mother tincture' used in herbal medicine is 10% solution. This is the first step in creating a homeopathic remedy. If the substance is a mineral, then it is ground with sugar into a fine powder. One part of this tincture is then mixed with 99 parts of distilled water and then shaken vigorously (succussion). This is now called the 1c dilution. It is a 1/1,000 dilution, which is never used as a medicine, because it is considered too weak to have any medicinal effect. In the next step, one part of the 1c is taken and mixed with another ninety-nine parts of distilled water and succussed, creating a 2c dilution potency. This process is repeated four more times to create the 6c potency. A 6c dilution is also considered to be a 'weak dose', but, therapeutically, it can be taken by a patient up to four times a day. The 6c potency has one part of the original substance in ten thousand trillion parts of water.

The 30c potency means that 24 more dilutions are made to the 6c dilution and this new concentration is one part of the original substance in 1, followed by 60 zeros, parts of water. I.e. 1/100, (60 zeros).

The 30c dilution will have a medicinal effect for about one day in a very severe first aid or acute ailment and up to two weeks in a mildly acute or chronic illness.

The strongest homeopathic doses are much smaller concentrations such as a 200c potency. This means that there is one part of the original substance as a fraction of 1 followed by 400 zeros parts of water. This number is so small there is no name for it. This strength of remedy can be used if the 30c worked well but no longer has any effect.

There are also 1,000c (1M) and 10,000c (10M) dilutions. These dilutions are used when the 200c is no longer having the desired effect; as one dose of the 1M will last for months, and the illness that it is used for needs to have met various criteria in order to warrant such a far-reaching treatment program. In certain first aid situations a 1M can be very useful.

The paradox of smaller and smaller doses, which have stronger and stronger medicinal action, has unfortunately kept homeopathy out of mainstream scientific medicine because there is no method to measure what is left in the dilution.

One day, science will discover that these medicines do contain small particles of matter, or specific energetic frequencies. The reason that the smaller doses have greater effect is because they have the ability to pass through cell walls in order to reach the part of the cell that needs the medicine in a dose that is still effective and non-toxic.

For example, a common homeopathic remedy Natrum muriaticum is made from table salt – sodium chloride. This medicine has - with great success - often been used for seemingly hopeless chronic ailments such as migraine headaches. Even though she was using salt every day in her diet, the potentized remedy becomes unique in its healing effects, and acts differently than the crude substance.

In summary, the homeopathic remedies are very dilute solutions. They are thus non-toxic, but have the ability to stimulate homeostasis and a rapid healing reaction.

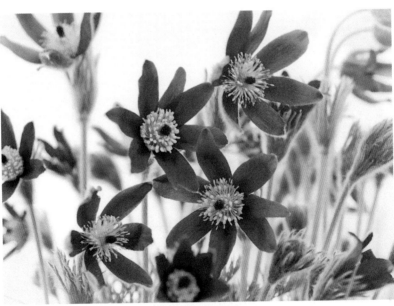

Pulsatilla Nigricans

How to administer the remedy

All homeopathic remedies are taken internally. (Arnica and Calendual 30c are taken like all other remedies, internally, but they also come in a cream to be used externally.)

Each remedy is available in liquid or granular form. There is no difference in the quality between the two. One dose of granules is 5 to 6 granules - let them dissolve under the tongue. If it is a liquid, shake it well by hitting the bottle on your palm at least ten times. Then take one teaspoon of the remedy in two table-spoons of water. Hold this solution under the tongue for about ten to thirty seconds to aid in its absorption before it is swallowed.

Do not eat or drink for fifteen minutes. This includes both before and after the liquid or granular remedy is taken. For the optimal effect, the remedy should be given as soon after the injury as possible. Take one dose in 30c potency. Often, this is all that is needed for an acute injury.

When to repeat or change the remedy

After one dose, there should be a positive change within ten minutes to 12 hours for a first aid ailment and 24 hours in the case of an acute illness. As long as improvement continues after this first dose then do not repeat the remedy. Repeat if symptoms begin to return or the improvement has obviously stopped.

There is no possibility of harm if the remedy is repeated when the symptoms begin to return. To gain the optimal effect of the remedy, it can also be repeated if some of the symptoms persist and there is no further improvement for one or two days in a row.

If there are no positive changes after the initial dose, do not repeat this first remedy choice. Look for more symptoms and try a second remedy. Repeating an incorrect remedy too often can lead to undesirable side effects. If the symptoms persist, consult a registered naturopath, professional homeopath or other medical professional.

In the case of very severe injuries, a higher strength of the remedy may be needed; such as a 200c potency. Use the 200c if the 30c has worked and helped. Do this (if after giving the 30c a few times) when there is no longer any effect and the condition of the patient is still the same. Only give one dose of the 200c potency and wait to see what the effect is. If it helps, then repeat it when there is a return of symptoms. A 1M is about four times stronger than the 200c and it too can be used if the 200c has no more effect. Repeat the 1M when symptoms return. In this manner, one can treat many conditions with homeopathy that one in the past would have had to use pain medications. Choose another remedy that is more strongly indicated if the first one is no longer effective and you have tried the first one in a higher potency.

ANTIDOTES: WHAT TO AVOID WHEN TAKING A REMEDY

Remedies may be antidoted (become ineffective) either partially or completely by various substances or other forms of treatment. Antidoting can greatly complicate treatment, therefore, it is essential to carefully avoid these influences. The following is a list of the more common ways in which the remedies can lose their effectiveness.

Caffeine – Coffee frequently antidotes remedies. The antidoting effect can occur after only one cup of coffee in some people or several cups of tea for another person. As there is no way to predict this, it is essential to avoid caffeine altogether.

Even after you feel much better and have stopped taking the remedy; it is important to not drink coffee or tea for a few days in the case for first aid, a few weeks in the case of an acute illness, and a few months in the case of a chronic illness. Water processed decaffeinated coffee (decaf coffee), caffeinated soft drinks and black tea also contain caffeine and should all be avoided. Some alternatives, which do not contain caffeine, are herbal teas, freeze dried decaffeinated coffee, hot chocolate and decaffeinated black tea. These are safe to drink and will ensure the effectiveness of the remedy. Chocolate is not an antidote in moderate amounts.

Camphor and other essential oils – Avoid anything that has camphor in it, such as deep heat liniments, Tiger Balm®, Vick's®, shaving cream with camphor, Noxzema® products, many lip balms, cough lozenges, essential oils such as eucalyptus, menthol, etc. A rub of camphorated oil, as well as long exposure to the odor itself, will antidote remedies. Essential oils are very useful for certain conditions, but unfortunately they will often antidote the remedy.

Allopathic drugs – Avoid antibiotics, cortisone, and over-the-counter pain medicines. These common drugs can suppress specific or local symptoms and weaken the patient. Therefore, these should be avoided except when prescribed by your medical provider and in an emergency or life-threatening condition.

Chemicals – Avoid paints, solvents, and sprays for pest and insect control, as these are known to antidote.

Electric blankets – Avoid the use of electric blankets (there appears to be a detrimental interaction of the electric field of the blanket with the body).

How to care for and handle the remedies

Store the remedy away from direct sunlight, electrical appliances and strong odors. Avoid placing it in a place where the temperature rises above eighty degrees Fahrenheit. A cool neutral environment; such as in a cupboard, alongside glass or paper products, is an ideal storage place.

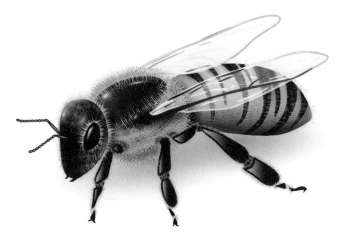

Apis Melifica

CHAPTER 2

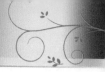

Homeopathy for Specific First Aid Conditions

For each condition you would like to treat, read all the remedies in each section, and select the ones that seem to cover all of your symptoms. Compare the ones that seem most likely. In the next book, **First Aid Mater Medica** - there is a further detailed explanation of many of these first aid remedies with case examples.

Not all the symptoms for each remedy are listed, as many of these remedies contain many common symptoms for that condition. I have, instead, listed the most frequently seen and unusual symptoms for each remedy.

Dosage: Take one dose of the 30c potency. *Repeat the dose only if the symptoms start to return,* or the progress stops. If the patient is recovering well and making progress, you do not need to repeat the remedy.

In a certain instance, such as a case of bleeding, the repetition of the dose may be needed after ten minutes if the bleeding starts up again. In the case of a cold, the person may need only one dose as they continue to improve by leaps and bounds every day. Each case is unique. Some cases are more severe and may need repeated doses, while some are mild and need fewer doses. One person may have a healing system that is very strong. Fewer doses would be needed. Others have a weaker constitution, and may need more frequent doses to stimulate it toward a cure.

The rule to follow is: Only repeat the dose when there is a relapse. This means the symptoms start to return, or the healing has stopped and won't progress past a certain point.

If healing is happening, (i.e., you see positive changes on a daily basis), then do not repeat the dose. There is no need, and it can actually slow down the progress in a person who is sensitive to that particular remedy.

Although I believe the 30c potency to be the best to use, you may only find a 6c potency or 12c potency available. In this case, you can still use these, but they may need to be repeated more often.

The 6c is the weakest dose and can be safely repeated three or four times a day. Next is the 12c that can be repeated two or three times a day. The 30c potency, which is still stronger, can be safely taken once a day to once a week depending on the severity of the illness. A 200c can usually be taken for a chronic illness once a month, but for a very severe acute illness, once a week. It is best to start with one dose of a 30c. If you have given it a few times and it no longer has any effect, then give a dose of 200c. If this is taken a few times and stops working, then take a 1m (1,000c).

I have abbreviated some of the names of the remedies. For example Aconite is actually Aconite napellus. There should not be any confusion when you purchase these remedies as the pharmacies use the same abbreviations.

ACCIDENTS – CAR – SEE Injuries

Use all necessary first aid measures that are available to you and that are at your skill level. Call 911 if there is any uncertainty to the severity of the injuries.

The main remedies to consider are as follows. You can read more about these remedies in the First Aid Materia Medica text.

Aconite 30c – For the FEAR, anxiety and symptoms of shock after a car accident. Disorientation and confusion from fear will be helped by Aconite. *Example:* After the plane crash, she had panic attacks. Aconite 30c helped this within an hour. After the car rolled over, her heart was beating forcefully, and she thought she was about to die. After a dose of Aconite, within five minutes, she felt calm. This remedy is indicated for sudden fear leading to rapid onset of symptoms.

Arnica 30c – TAKE FOR ANY INJURY or physical trauma when

there is pain experienced in any part of the body after a car accident. This remedy is indicated for the general trauma when there is bruised soreness from the injury. It can be used to stop bleeding and heal bruises. Works best for sore bruised muscles and joints; sprained ankles and sports injuries; before and after surgery. *Example:* After the fall down the stairs, she was crying from the bump on her head. After giving birth, the baby had a bruise on the head. After playing golf, his back was so painful he could not tie his shoes.

Bryonia 30c – Useful for injuries after a car accident where

the pain is worse from any motion. At rest there is almost no pain but on motion of the affected area the pain can be intense. For example, after the injury the neck is stiff and painfully worse from any motion. Even a slight movement of the head would cause a sharp pain. Take one dose of a 30c. Repeat if the pain returns.

Ledum pulustra 30c – Trauma with pain to soft tissues and

nerves. This past summer I closed a car door on my index finger. The pain was extreme – I felt it through my whole body and it even made me feel depressed. The fingernail filled with blood almost right away. As it was better from cold applications, I took Ledum 30c, and almost immediately the pain abated. I felt overall better. Ledum is also listed to treat trauma to the finger tips and resulting nerve pain (pain neuralgic: Ledum).

Carbo animalis 30c – Use for *mental dullness after a car accident*. **Take for** WEAKNESS of the muscles after an injury or weakness that is worse from lifting. For example, after lifting the grocery bags to the car, she felt totally exhausted for the rest of the day. This is sometimes noticed days or weeks after the injury. Take Arnica first after an injury to the head. If this has helped, try Arnica 200c to see if any more benefit can be gained from the Arnica. If not, then consider Carbo-an.

Cocculus 30c – Use for vertigo after a head injury. She can't concentrate, in a fog, neck is weak and sore. There may be nausea with the vertigo. Feeling dizzy and light headed. *In reference to the nausea, the smell of food makes the nausea feel worse. In later stages, there may be weakness all over the body, mental confusion, severe vertigo and nausea. This remedy is treating the nerves and muscles.*

Helleborus 30c – Can use after a car accident or has been hit on the head. May have concussion (the *mind is very slow to respond)*. There is a long delay after you ask this person a question. This remedy can be used after a head injury or concussion when the mind becomes very slow. The mind is physically deteriorating. There is a delay in answering questions. The memory is very poor. There may be an emotional depression as well.

Hypericum 30c – Head injury, trauma to *nerve tissue*. Sharp pains in the head, neck or down the arms. Arnica is for any type of pain so it is best to take it first. If, after the Arnica, there are sharp shooting pains, lightning pains, or the pain that one can imagine from having a nerve squeezed, then try Hypericum 30c (one dose).

Rhus-tox 30c – Use when the main symptom is STIFFNESS . May use if there is stiffness of the neck, back or joint. *The stiffness will be worse when starting to move and better from continued motion.* The stiffness is also worse from cold damp weather and better from a hot bath or shower. If the injury is very recent, this symptom may not be noticeable. If Arnica has done what it can and stiffness is still a major symptom, then Rhus tox may be the next remedy to try. Take 30c (one dose) and wait a few days to evaluate its effect.

ANAPHYLAXIS –

A sudden allergic reaction where there is difficulty in breathing. Call 911, as this condition can be life threatening.

Apis 30c – Can be used for allergy and anaphylaxis. The skin is red, swollen, and worse from heat. There may be difficulty breathing because of an allergic influence. *Example:* After a bee sting, his face was swollen, and he experienced breathing difficulties. Shellfish, peanuts and medications are other triggers for anaphylaxis. Apis can be employed. I have seen this remedy work for a patient who was allergic to adrenalin. When the ambulance arrived, they were thankful that there was an alternative to the usual treatment for anyphylaxis.

ANIMAL BITES – INCLUDING SCRATCHES –

Depending on the severity of the wound, you may need to consult a physician. You may also be in need of a tetanus shot.

Calendula 30c – This remedy can be taken internally for any kind of animal scratch or bite. Also, apply Calendula cream to the surface of the wound. (Calendula cream or ointment are also available for external use.) Calendula stimulates the immune system to kill bacteria and viruses. I have never seen a wound become infected after Calendula was applied to it. For deeper infections, after a wound or surgery, the 30c is needed. For very severe infections, it may be needed a few times a day (to save a person's life). Use once every three days after surgery to prevent infections from developing. If the 30c has helped, but not cured the case, then use Calendula 200c and repeat when symptoms return.

Ledum 30c – Use for sore, swollen wounds caused from bites or from stepping on a sharp object (such as a nail). Ledum is most useful for mosquito bites, but it can also be used after any type of animal bite to prevent infection. It can prevent a lymphatic infection where one can see a blue streak extending further and further up the limb. Another name for this condition is lymphangitis. The itching of the mosquito bite feels better after putting ice on it.

Hypericum 30c – Useful for any animal bite toxin introduced into the soft tissues of the body. Especially useful if the pain is sharp or shooting in nature.

Supportive treatment: Clean the wound as best you can. One can also apply a paste of Activated Charcoal on a wound which can help to keep it clean.

ANXIETY – FROM PHYSICAL TRAUMA –

After an accident, fear and anxiety are often a result.

Aconite 30c – This is a routine remedy to take after any injury or car accident that produces SUDDEN ANXIETY or FEAR of DEATH. Often, after an accident, there are panic and fear thoughts and feelings. There may be an idea that something awful could have happened. After a car accident the person is in shock. They feel disorientated. They may have a glazed look in their eyes. They may be breathing too rapidly and feel faint with a racing heart. They may feel restless anxiety after a fright or after an injury. They may be crying with the anxiety.

ANTICIPATION ANXIETY – STAGE FRIGHT –

This fear takes place before an important event such as a job interview or before a performance.

Gelsemium 30c – This is for anticipation anxiety. Take *for fear and anxiety before an important event*, accompanied by increased heart rate, *trembling*, and a FEAR OF FAILURE.

Examples:
- He was very anxious about his job interview. He was so anxious that he did not want to leave his house.
- She was nervous she wouldn't pass her exam. The nervousness made her forget all she had learned.

This remedy can be used for fear and anxiety before a stage performance. Take one dose of Gelsemium 30c when the anxiety starts. Most likely that is all that will be needed. Useful for weakness and forgetfulness from anxiety.

Lycopodium 30c – Useful for fear before an event, such as, being on stage, an exam, or a job interview. The abdomen feels bloated and tired upon waking in the morning. May compensate to the fear by being aggressive toward others. A person may have an overall lack of confidence, with a desire to avoid the situation.

BACK PAIN –
I have used all of these remedies for back pain and seen how well they can work when they are given when the symptoms agree.

Arnica 30c – Useful if *sore and achy in the muscles (from over-lifting or from trauma to the back, such as a sports injury or car accident).* May feel like a FAILURE or feel "good for nothing." Can be used after the loss of job or loss of financial security with back pain. If the back injury has just occurred, then this remedy should be taken first to heal the bruising. After a back injury, he had to walk bent forward, and could not touch his toes or bend backward. Back pains worsen from touch or pressure.

Bambusa 30c – Useful for *very stiff, rigid muscles* in the back and neck. Muscles in the back are in spasm, rigid and so stiff that he can't turn his head or bend forward or bend the neck to the side. Could be from over lifting, a fall or from some other trauma. Often feel they need help from others; that they need to do everything one hundred and ten percent. Displays extreme perfectionist behavior. She folds her dirty laundry before washing it. She wants help and support in her life but can't find it. I, personally, have used this remedy with success for a very painful back spasm.

Hypericum 30c – For injuries to the spine or head. May have sharp or shooting pains. May have numbness. May be worse from foggy weather.

Nux-vomica 30c – Useful for tension in the back, spasmodic muscles. For people who can't relax, *ambitious, impatient, fastidious* (angry from disorder), and hard working. Useful if sensitive to cold and drafts on the back. Condition gets worse from noise. May like coffee but you need to abstain from all caffeine for a few months when taking the remedy. Take one dose of the 30c every seven to ten days until you feel 95% better. Here is a famous quote describing the Nux temperament: "Is the greatest of polychrests (a remedy with many uses), because the bulk of its symptoms correspond in similarity with those of the most common and most frequent of diseases.

…Nux is pre-eminently the remedy for many of the conditions incident to modern life. The typical Nux patient is rather thin, spare, quick, active, nervous, and irritable. He does a good deal of mental work; has mental strains and leads a sedentary life, found in prolonged office work, overstudy, and close application to business, with its cares and anxieties. This indoor lifestyle and mental strain seeks stimulants, coffee, wine, possibly in excess; or, again, he hopes to quiet his excitement, by indulging in the sedative effects of tobacco, if not really a victim to the seductive drugs, like opium, etc.

These things are associated with other indulgences. At the table, he takes preferably rich and stimulating food; wine and women play their part to make him forget the close application of the day. Late hours are a consequence; a thick head, dyspepsia, and irritable temper are the next day's inheritance. Now he takes some cathartic, liver pills, or mineral water, and soon gets into the habit of taking these things, which still further complicate matters.

Since these frailties are more yielded to by men than women, Nux is pre-eminently a male remedy. These conditions produce an IRRITABLE, nervous system, hypersensitive and over impressionable, which Nux will do much to soothe and calm. Especially adapted to digestive disturbances, portal congestion, and hypochondrical states depending thereon. Convulsions, with consciousness; worse, touch, moving. ZEALOUS FIERY TEMPERAMENT. Nux patients are easily chilled, avoid open air, etc. Nux always seems to be out of tune; inharmonious spasmodic action."
– Materia Medica by Boericke

Rhus tox 30c – STIFF back *(especially after sitting or on waking in the morning)*. Better from a hot shower or from gentle exercise or from walking for half an hour. Worse from cold damp weather.

Ruta 30c – Pain in the back at night. Old back injuries or from *overuse of the back*, such as construction work. May have excessive guilt over small incidents. He or she is too conscientious. May feel anxiety in a warm closed-in room.

Bee Stings –
These remedies can also be used for wasp stings and spider bites.

Ledum – For bites and puncture wounds, infected wounds and especially mosquito bites. *Example:* The bite produced a large itchy lump.

Apis 30c – For bites that swell up, itch or feel warm. Bites that progress to an allergic response or even to anaphylaxis. Skin is red, swollen and worse from heat. Difficulty with breathing because of an allergic influence. *Example:* After a bee sting his face was swollen, and he experienced breathing difficulties. Give a dose of Apis 30c and call 911.

BITES – SEE Insect bites OR Bee Stings
These remedies can be helpful for insect bites and stings.

BLEEDING FROM TRAUMA –
Use all usual first aid measures along with the indicated remedy. If in doubt as to the extent of the injuries call 911.

Arnica 30c – *Bleeding from trauma,* bruising and pain. Useful for head injury, concussion. Use this remedy first. Repeat the dose only when the symptoms return. Take one dose before and after any surgery.

Calendula 30c – *For any open wound* this remedy can be taken to help stop the bleeding, prevent infection, and help to close the wound. Take one dose before and after any surgery to prevent excessive bleeding. It is okay to take Arnica 30c and then an hour later take a dose of Calendula 30c. For minor cuts this remedy can be applied as a cream to the wound, then covered with a band-aid.

Bellis perennis 30c – Especially indicated for pelvic injuries. Use after trauma or surgery to deep organs of the body. Injuries to the bladder or uterus, especially. There may be pain in the pelvis on exertion or a sensation of swelling and tenderness in the pelvic area. The first remedy to use after any pelvic or abdominal surgery.

Ficus religiosa 30c – For *bleeding that is very extensive* and threatens the person's life after an injury. If Arnica 30c is not helping, you can try a stronger dose of Arnica, such as Arnica 200c or Arnica 1m. Try this remedy if Arnica keeps relapsing or seems ineffective.

Ipecacuanha 30c – For excessive *bleeding that is accompanied by nausea.* Sometimes this happens after surgery or after childbirth.

Millifolium 30c – For sore wounds and bleeding wounds. May be bright red blood.

BONES INJURIES –
For broken bones, bruised bones.

Symphytum 30c – This remedy is very useful for bone injuries. Can be used for bruised or broken bones or pain in the bone from an injury.
Examples:
- He knocked his shin on a concrete park bench.
- He hit his finger with a hammer and bruised the bone.
- Her jaw hurt after the dental surgery.
- After a hit on the head, the scalp was very sore to touch.
- It can also be used for softening of bones.

Calcarea-phos 30c – May have pain in the bones or tendons after an injury. The lower limbs feel restless and want to move. There may be lameness and weakness. Cramps in the calves may be present. Growing pains may occur. Bones may be soft in parts and develop caries (cavitations).

BRAIN AND HEAD TRAUMA – SEE Head Injury AND Car Accidents

It is best to receive an evaluation done by a health professional after a head injury. But also take Arnica to begin with and/or consult a homeopathic practitioner.

Arnica 30c – Take this first. It can prevent bleeding of the brain, aid in symptoms of concussion, and help the person regain consciousness. Repeat the dose when symptoms return.

Hypericum 30c – For shooting or sharp pains in the head.

Cicuta 30c – For convulsions after a head injury.

Cocculus indicus 30c – For nausea after a head injury, vertigo and the thinking processes have become obviously slow. The head feels very heavy. The mind feels dull.

Burns –

The immediate pain of a burn can be treated with cold water. Fresh Aloe Vera gel (a mucilaginous substance from breaking the stem of this plant and applying it directly on the burned area) has a reputation in helping burn pain.

Cantharis 30c – *For burns from fire, heat or hot water.* Use for PAIN and BLISTERING from a burn. Examples: The child touched the hot wood stove and the skin burned. The boiling water from the kettle blistered his fingers. The fire scorched his back. Use for work related burns from hot machinery. It is unfortunate that the prejudice against homeopathy has kept this remedy from being used in all hospitals to treat burns.

I have never seen Cantharis fail to stop the pain of a burn in a matter of seconds or minutes. If the burn is very severe and the 30c potency does not bring continued relief, then use the 200c potency. If after three doses this continues to relapse, then try the 1m potency or even a dose of the 10m potency.

Causticum 30c – This is known to help chemical burns.

Urtica urens 30c – This remedy can be used for sun burn or tried if Cantharis has no or only a minimal effect.

CAR ACCIDENTS –

The effects of a car accident can affect many different tissues of the body, such as muscle, tendons, ligaments and/or the deeper organs of the body. Have an evaluation by a chiropractor and your physician. Below are listed the most commonly used remedies.

Aconite 30c – For the *fear and anxiety which occurs immediately following a car accident.* Useful for shock symptoms after a car accident and/or disorientation.

Arnica 30c – Take this first for the general trauma. Use for bruised sore pains all over. Also, useful to stop any bleeding.

Bryonia 30c – For pain that is worse from motion (even very slight motion).

Carbo animalis 30c – Useful for mental dullness after a car accident. Take for weakness that is worse from lifting or carrying things.

Cocculus 30c – For vertigo or nausea after a head injury. She can't concentrate, is in a fog, neck is weak and sore.

Hypericum 30c – For head injury and/or trauma to nerve tissue. Useful for sharp pains.

Rhus-tox 30c – Use when the main symptom is stiffness.

Symphytum 30c – For bruising to bones or trauma to tendons or ligaments. Pains may be worse at night. Good for old spinal injuries.

CRAMPS – SEE Muscle Trauma

Often, this is a chronic tendency, which will need a chronic remedy like Calcarea carbonica or Magnesia carbonica. It is best to consult a registered homeopathic doctor for this.

CUTS AND SCRAPES –
These are some of the most common type of ailments, especially for children. Clean the wound as best you can, then take Calendula as directed below.

Calendula 30c – For pain from an injury to the skin. This remedy prevents wound infection. It is indicated for any cuts and scrapes. Use for cellulitis (infected tissues) from surgery. *Example:* The finger was cut with a knife. Recommendation: Calendula ointment applied and bandaged. Calendula 30c may be taken orally to strengthen the immune system and prevent infection.

Calendula cream – Use on the wound externally.

DENTAL WORK REMEDIES –

Painful dentition –

Topics below:
  • Fear before a dental appointment

- Pain and to prevent infection (take before or after)
- Infection or for a dental abscess or infection of the nerve root
- Tooth ache
- Hemorrhage after surgery
- Systemic infection

FEAR BEFORE A DENTAL APPOINTMENT –

Aconite 30c – For fear of going to see the dentist. The person gets heart palpitations, rapid breathing before dental treatment. Take one dose the day before the appointment. Compare this remedy to Gelsemium and Lycopodium. Look in the section: Anticipation Anxiety.

Gelsemium – For fear of dental work. Take a dose the day before the appointment. He or she may experience diarrhea, trembling, weakness or even get flu-like symptoms before the appointment. This is similar to the feeling of stage fright.

PAIN AND TO PREVENT INFECTION BEFORE OR AFTER SURGERY –

Arnica 30c – Take one dose before and after dental surgery. It will prevent bleeding and pain.

Calendula 30c - Use before and after dental surgery to prevent pain and infection. Calendula is the great WOUND healer and can be used in conditions that arise after INCISIONS and CUTS to the gums.

Calendula is also the medicine of choice for any SURGERY or operation on any part of the body. It will prevent INFECTION and stimulate rapid healing of the skin and underlying tissues. Give 30c every two days for one week after the surgery.

Hypericum 30c – Take this before surgery to prevent *pain* *to the tooth nerve root.* This remedy can be taken an hour or two before the appointment to prevent nerve pain or after the appointment for the same.

I am one of the 99% of the population that does not normally look forward to going to the dentist. Anything that can make the experience less traumatic has to be helpful.

A few years ago I had an old filling loosen, and the tooth became painful. On examination, it was found that a deeper cavity had formed under the old amalgam filling. "A simple procedure," said the dentist, "we will just take out the old filling, drill out the decay and put in a new filling." I asked if my mouth would have to be frozen and he said, "Definitely, as the cavity was deep and the drill would likely affect the nerve of the tooth, causing considerable pain."

For the past few years, I had been teaching courses on how to use homeopathy for common ailments. One of the medicines I always mentioned is called Hypericum perforatum 30c. It is made from a tincture of St. Johns Wort.

It is used in homeopathic doses for pain that arises after an injury to a nerve. Specifically, it treats the electric and sharp shooting types of pain. This is seen in situations of having the fingers or toes crushed, biting of one's tongue, a spinal injury or dental treatment.

"Now this is a situation where I should be able to take a few doses of Hypericum and not have to use any anesthetic", I thought to myself. On making this proposal to the dentist, he assured me, "this drilling is going to cause you a lot of pain and was I really sure only taking the Hypericum was a good idea?"

I took one dose of the Hypericum 30c and waited a few minutes, and then he started to drill. He kept asking me, "Are you okay?" and I kept assuring him that there was no pain. He used a sharp drill and then one that felt more coarse or "bumpy" but all seemed to be going well. Then I felt one of those pains he had mentioned. It was like an electric shock!

I took another dose of the Hypericum 30c, waited a few minutes and then he finished the drilling with no recurrence of the pain. The cavity was filled; I thanked him for letting me do a test with Hypericum.

I would recommend you use Hypericum 30c, 4 to 6 granules a half hour before the dental treatment that involves drilling. It is up to you to also take the usual anesthetic. This remedy could be especially helpful if you happen to be one of those people who is not anesthetized easily by dental anesthetic, or you are allergic to dental anesthetic.

Symphytum 30c – This remedy can be used when there has been *trauma to the bones of the jaw.* Use for pain that is from surgery or bruising of the periosteum (the living tissue around the bone). Especially, if the dentist is going to cut into the bone, then Symphytum will be needed. Tooth extractions will also benefit from it, as the bone is traumatized by this procedure. For bones that are weak and break easily, take one dose every two weeks for three months.

INFECTION OR FOR A DENTAL ABSCESS OR INFECTION TO THE NERVE ROOT –

Belladonna 30c – For a dental abscess, infected socket in the initial stages. Use when there is pulsating pain and/or throbbing pains. There may be a dry fever, redness of the gum and the eyes become sensitive to light.

Hepar sulph 30c – For abscesses in the gums or roots of the teeth. Especially if the person is very sensitive to cold and can't get warm again easily.

Merc sol or merc viv 30c – Useful if the gums are spongy, bleed, and the roots are easily infected. This is another deep acting medicine for severe and chronic infections of the ears and other organs. There are so many excellent symptoms to indicate the use of Merc-sol. It should not be difficult to prescribe.

These symptoms include *sensitivity to hot and cold.* The patient will find it difficult to find a comfortable temperature – the room either feels too warm or too chilly. The person seems to take on the character of mercury itself: When it is hot, they feel too warm; when it is cold, they feel too chilled. The patient can't maintain their resistance to hot and cold. For example, when the bed gets hot she throws off the covers. Then she feels a chill so turns up the heat. Then she breaks out in a cold sweat and has to open the window. Not many remedies have this symptom, so when it is present, it becomes a super keynote for Mercury.

SALIVATION ON THE PILLOW WHEN SLEEPING
Wakes up in the morning with wet spots on the pillow.

SWOLLEN CERVICAL GLANDS
The lymphatic glands of the neck are puffy and hardened. This is a common symptom in chronic infections of the upper respiratory tract (bronchi, throat, nasal passages) and/or a tooth abscess.

PERSPIRATION AT NIGHT WHICH AGGRAVATES
Often, will experience a cold and clammy sweat all over the body. It can be a profuse, heavy sweat. It does not bring relief of any symptoms, and the person will say, "I feel worse from it."

PALE, SICKLY LOOKING
The face can be swollen and moist. Might have pale, white skin, sunken eyes, dark around the eyes and dry lips. The tongue is swollen, coated white, and showing the imprint of the teeth.

SYMPTOMS WORSE AT NIGHT
Bone pains, fever, ear pains, sleeplessness, cough, sore throat, all can be worse at night.

EFFECTS OF INFECTION SUCH AS, PUS FORMATION, ABSCESSES,

ULCERATIONS
Use Merc-sol 30c when all or most of these symptoms are present:

- Thick mucous from the sinuses, thick yellow discharge from the ears

- Boils in the ear canals

- Swollen tonsils with pus and bad breath

- Bronchitis and pneumonia with heavy tough mucous that is difficult to cough up

- Ulcers of the mouth and throat

Silica 30c – For abscesses on the gums or in the roots of the teeth. This remedy is able to cure very deep, chronic, infectious tendencies.

At least some of the following general and keynote symptoms of Silica have to be present in order for the remedy to be the simillimum. Simillimum is the word we use to describe the exact remedy that is needed for a patient.

- Sensitive to cold, to a draft, or cold and heat, but not just an aggravation from heat

- Sensitive to cold, with cold hands and feet

- Easy perspiration on the feet and the head

- Perspiration of the head during sleep (Calcarea carbonica also has this symptom.)

- Hypersensitive to noise

- Constipation, or a hard stool (Most people that need Silica have some sort of constipation problem.)

- Nervous weakness

- Variable thirst

- Aggravation from milk

- Ingrown toe nails

- White spots on the nails of the hands

TOOTH ACHE –

Hypericum 30c – Useful for shooting pains in the gums or jaw.

Plantago major 30c – Useful for toothache, decayed teeth, infected socket. Also good for neuralgic pains and if sensitive to touch. Use if teeth feel too long. Helps if worse from cold air. The toothache feels better while eating. Use if have symptom of profuse flow of saliva and/or dirty taste in the mouth. Can be used locally on the tooth.

HEMORRHAGE AFTER SURGERY –

Arnica 30c – Take this first. It will most likely take care of the bleeding. Repeat the 30c dose if the bleeding starts up again.

Calendula 30c – Take this to stop the bleeding and to prevent pain and infection.

Phosphorus 30c – Try a dose of this remedy if the Arnica is of no help. A strong thirst for cold drinks calls for this remedy.

SYSTEMIC INFECTIONS –

Calendula 30c – This will usually prevent any infection if it is taken the day before oral surgery, and then a dose right after the surgery.

Pyrogen 30c – To prevent bacterial infections any place in the body after surgery, such as endocarditis (infection of the heart muscle). Usually the dentist will prescribe antibiotics. If these have not helped you in the past, or you are allergic to antibiotics, then you can take this remedy to prevent infection. If any infection symptoms appear, see your doctor or consult a professional homeopath.

I gave this to a patient one time, who would get blood poisoning every time his body received a cut or even a scrape. He was a carpenter. Even though he was very careful, he would still, at times, injure himself. On the occasion I saw him, he had scraped his leg. The whole leg had become infected, plus he had a fever. His doctor suggested he have his leg amputated as the antibiotics were not helping him. He protested saying, "If I lose my leg, how am I going to work?" I gave him some doses of Pyrogen 30c. He healed up without any more complications. From then on, he no longer was prone to infections from cuts and scrapes.

Dislocation to the elbow or shoulder –
Seek out a physician to mobilize the joint back into position.

Hypericum 30c – Numbness and tingling of the arm after a dislocation. This remedy can be used any time a nerve has been stretched.

Earthquakes – see also Natural Disasters
This type of event naturally produces a lot of fear. Take Arnica 30c if there is any bruising. Look to the other sections in this book, such as Injuries, for the effects of injuries.

Aconite 30c – *Sudden shock leading to a fear of death.* The building fell down right beside her. She thought she was about to die and was filled with anxiety.

Eye strain –
This often happens from reading computer monitors or in a

work situation that requires a lot of close eye work.

Ruta 30c – *For eye pain from overuse of the eyes.* This remedy can also be used for tendinitis from over-use of a joint. *Pain from repetitive use and also when at rest.* Examples: After working all day bagging groceries, her wrists ached. His job as an editor required reading text off a computer terminal leading to eye strain. At night his eyes ached and felt very tired. She had to stop the heavy golf schedule because of the pain in her elbow.

FALLS – SEE ALSO Injuries

Arnica 30c – For pain from physical trauma. Use for muscle injury, joint sprain, black and blue bruises. Examples: A sprained ankle or a child who falls and bruises her head.

Hypericum 30c – Sharp pains and from stretching of a nerve.

Rhus tox 30c – For stiffness and pain in any joint after an injury. *Use for pain that improves with heat and motion.* *Example:* After the car accident, her back was very stiff, especially after sitting and after sleeping. She felt worse when she first began to move but improved with continued motion, and after taking a hot shower.

FEAR AND ANXIETY FROM PHYSICAL TRAUMA –
Often after an injury, fear and anxiety are present. If this symptom is present, the following remedies can be of great benefit.

Aconite 30c – For any shock that produces fear and trembling. *Use for sudden fear of death from a near-death experience.* The body feels cold. Panic and traumatic feelings are experienced. *Example:* After a car accident, she went into shock. Useful for palpitations of the heart.

Arnica 30c – Feels in shock after a trauma. Useful if experiencing nightmares after physical trauma.

FEAR OF DEATH FROM TRAUMA –

Aconite 30c – Anxiety that comes on suddenly. *Take a dose after any life threatening situation.* The fear of death remains long after the accident or initial trauma.

Arnica 30c – Helpful if one feels shaken up after a fright. The mind is sluggish when in shock. Helpful if sore all over from the trauma. Use if one feels beaten down after a severe economic shock. One may have feelings like they have failed in life and become useless (such as a depression that comes on from being unemployed).

Opium 30c – After a trauma, the person is full of fear. They are either falling asleep in the daytime or can't sleep at night or both. May go into shock and feel dissociated from their feelings. May have snoring, sleep apnea and/or obstinate constipation. May feel dreamy and drowsy in the daytime. May have difficulty telling the truth; lying for no reason. Ailments that are usually painful are not, but rather numb or painless.

FEAR FROM ANTICIPATION –
Before an event, the person feels fear, lack of confidence and/or panic.

Aconite 30c – Can use this for fear of death or fear that something terrible will happen before an event. Can use Aconite 30c for fear to fly in an airplane or for fear of going through a tunnel. The fear can be so severe; it leads to a full-blown panic attack. This is a quick acting remedy. You should feel better (in a matter of minutes) after taking only one dose.

Argentum nitricum 30c – Use for fear of all types of things, but especially a fear of going over a bridge, flying in an airplane or being on stage. Useful for *many irrational fears* because the imagination in these type of people is overactive and they can always think of the worst thing that could happen.

"If I get the surgery – this could cause an infection, then blood poisoning and then I will die – then who will look after my children – and then some bad thing could then happen to them – what if they are kidnapped? – and so it goes ..."

These patients have a strong fear of closed spaces. There are symptoms of craving for sweets and salt. In general, he feels worse from eating sweets. Can have fear with palpitations. Can have lots of bloating and loud belching. Can be very extroverted people with a good sense of humor, i.e., they can think up lots of funny ideas.

Gelsemium 30c – Useful for symptoms of trembling before going to an event or an appointment. Useful for a weakness of the legs, mental confusion, and difficulty speaking (from fear). Use if one can't write an exam, can't perform the recital, can't go to the dentist and/or feels cowardly. Use if the patient feels as though they want to run away from stress.

Lycopodium 30c – Fear before an event. Upset stomach, gas and bloating. Finds excuse not to go. Feels inadequate to the task at hand. Fear of new things and new people. Dictatorial and controlling of others. Wakes unrefreshed in the morning. May have an aggravation from eating onions, oysters, and spicy food. Eating ever so little causes fullness in the abdomen. They act confident on the surface but deeper down they feel fear.

Food Poisoning –
Often this happens while traveling. Take these remedies with you on your next trip. Although, there are many homeopathic pharmacies in foreign countries.

Arsenicum album 30c and Veratrum album 30c –

Both can be used for food poisoning (bacterial gastritis), nausea, chills, *vomiting and/ or diarrhea* caused by unclean food or water. Recommendation: Take Arsenicum 30c first. If this does not help within a few hours, then take Veratrum album 30c. Only take Veratrum 30c first, if the diarrhea happens at the same time as the vomiting.

Carbo vegetabilis 30c – Nausea and/or vomiting. Take when

the body feels lifeless and cold, but patient wants fresh air or to be fanned. Bloated in the abdomen but feels a little better from belching. Worse from eating fats.

Also look at the section on Nausea.

HEAD INJURY –

Consult a physician for this condition to rule out any serious effect of the injury. If none of these remedies fails to describe your symptoms, then find a professional homeopath. Also look at the section on "Injuries –" on page 51.

Arnica 30c – Take this first for pain and/or bruising on the head.

Cocculus indicus 30c – Take this if there is vertigo or

nausea after the head injury. Nausea or *vertigo is worse from missing a good night's sleep.* Inability to concentrate.

Hypericum 30c – Take this if there are any shooting pains or neck injury.

Natrum sulphur 30c – Take this if there is a depression after the head injury.

Cicuta virosa 30c – Take if there are any twitches or convulsions after the head injury.

Helleborus 30c – Take if there is depression or the person is *slow to answer questions* after the head injury.

HYPERVENTILATION –

In this condition, the person would have most likely experienced a fright. The breathing becomes too rapid and fainting can result.

Aconite 30c – After a car accident or a natural disaster, there may be a feeling of shock. The patient may have frequent breaths that leave the person feeling as if they will soon faint.

INFLAMED WOUNDS – SEE ALSO Wounds AND Puncture

WOUNDS –

This is the same remedy we use for all cuts and scrapes. Consult a physician if a wound has become infected.

Use **Calendula 30c** internally and apply Calendula cream to the wound.

Hypericum 30c – For any wound that has affected a nerve. Usually there are sharp shooting pains.

Ledum 30c – For any wound that feels cold or may have some animal poison in it.

INJURIES –

Such as sports injuries, car accidents, work-related injuries, falls, sprains, and birth trauma.

Arnica 30c – This is the first remedy to take for any injury.

Take this for pain from *any physical trauma.* Use for sports injury, falls, sprains and bruises.

Ledum 30c – Useful for sore swollen joints, relief gained from cold applications.

Rhus tox 30c – Useful for older injuries which are stiff and sore. The stiffness worsens when beginning motion and feels better when motion is continued. Pain gets better with heat but worse with cold and damp weather.

Ruta 30c – For old injuries like tendinitis, pain at night or when at rest. Pain is worse from overuse of the joint.

Bryonia 30c – Pain worse from any motion. It is better when kept perfectly still.

Symphytum 30c – Injuries to bones, bruised bones, broken bones, black eyes.

Carbo animalis 30c – Injuries that lead to a weakness after lifting or weakness after use of the arm, neck/back or legs. Pain and weakness from overuse of an injured joint.

INSECT BITES – SEE ALSO Animal bites **AND** Bee Stings

Ledum 30c – For bites from *mosquitoes* or another insect or animal. Bites which cause swelling, infection, itching, or aching. I have given this to people who seem to be allergic to mosquito bites. Good for mosquito bites that persist for weeks after the bite and don't seem to stop itching. It is a wonder how well it can heal this condition.

Apis 30c – Bites that lead to allergy symptoms, such as heat, itching and swelling.

JOINT INJURIES – SEE ALSO Injuries
Depending on the severity of the injury, you may need to see a health professional.

Arnica 30c – Try this first. If one dose does not help within 12 to 24 hours, then try one of the other remedies.

Carbo animalis 30c – Weakness of the joint and limb after an injury.

Bryonia 30c – For joint injury. Pain is worse from any motion and never better with motion. Feels better when kept very still. *Example:* After the injury to the wrist, he had to keep it very still or else, if he moved it, ever so slightly, the pain was very sharp.

Rhus tox 30c – Stiffness is the main symptom.

Ruta 30c – Old injuries that, after months, will not heal. Pain worse at night. Often these people, for some reason, feel unnecessarily guilty. Their conscience is too strong.

Symphytum 30c – Tearing of cartilage and ligaments. The pain will often be worse at night. Pulled tendons or ligaments. Loose joints after an injury.

MOTION SICKNESS –
The middle ear can often not adjust to the motion of cars, airplanes and boats. Nausea, dizziness and vomiting can result.

Cocculus 30c – Nausea and dizzy from riding in a car. The nausea is worse from the smell of cooking food.

Tabacum 30c – Nausea with icy cold body and perspiration; relief from exposing the body or abdomen to cool air. The motion sickness is better from opening the car window.

Petroleum 30c – Nausea with excessive saliva.

MUSCLE TRAUMA, CRAMPS, STRAINS, BRUISES –
Bruises, pain from sports injuries, after a car accident, after a fall.

Arnica 30c – First remedy to take for any injury. Pain from trauma. Use for sports injury, falls, sprains and bruises.

Ledum 30c – Sore swollen joints. *Relief is gained from cold applications.*

Rhus tox 30c – Older injuries which are stiff and sore. Stiffness is worse when beginning motion and better when motion is continued. The pain is better with heat, but worse with cold and damp weather.

Ruta 30c – Old injuries like tendinitis. Use for symptoms of pain at night or when at rest and worse from overuse.

Bryonia 30c – Pain worse from any motion but better when kept perfectly still.

Symphytum 30c – Injuries to bones, bruised bones, broken bones and black eyes.

Carbo animalis 30c – Use after an injury when there is weakness. Use for weakness after lifting of the arm, neck or legs. Pain and weakness from overuse of an injured joint. Worse from any exertion.

NATURAL DISASTERS –
Earthquakes, floods and/or any other sudden threat to life.

Arnica 30c – For *pain after the injury.*

Aconite 30c – For the fear after the injury. Useful for panic attacks and *rapid heart beat.*

Arsenicum 30c – For fear of lost family and possessions after the injury. Patient has a feeling of panic and insecurity. The person will become *meticulous.* They want order and have a desire to keep things *very neat* and clean. Sensitive and worse from cold or becoming chilled.

NAUSEA – MOTION SICKNESS – CAR, BOAT, AIRPLANE –
These are the most commonly used remedies for this condition. These remedies can also be used for nausea during pregnancy.

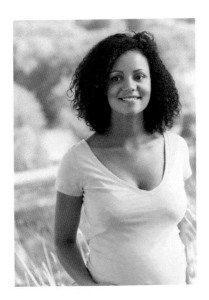

Cocculus is indicated if the nausea is accompanied by dizziness and/or is worse from the smell of food.

Tabacum is indicated when nausea is accompanied with a desire to expose the abdomen to cold air. The nausea feels better if the person can sit outside in the cool open air.

Petroleum is indicated when nausea is accompanied by excessive saliva. *Example:* After twenty minutes in the car, she felt nauseous.

Nerve Injuries –

Hypericum 30c – For nerve injury with shooting pain. Examples: After the car accident, she felt a shooting pain from her back into her arms. After hitting his finger with the hammer, he had shooting pain up his arm. Nerves are often injured if there are lightning pains or numbness.

Allium cepa 30c – Phantom limb pain after an amputation.

Overuse Injuries –
Tendons, ligamental strains and chronic inflammation.

Ruta 30c – For old injuries that are painful at night. Worse from any use of the affected area.

Symphytum 30c – For old injuries to joints. Symptoms feel worse from overuse. This remedy strengthens tendons, ligaments and cartilages. Weakness of the joint affected. Sometimes you can find this remedy prepared as a paste in a health food store. It is often mixed with olive oil or bees wax. This is a good way to take it externally, and can be rubbed into the affected joint at night before going to sleep. *Example:* Her knee was sore from training for a marathon; after rubbing on the Comfrey paste (Symphytum), she felt the knee was more stable and there was less pain.

Pain –
A quick reference for remedies that treat different types of pain

Arnica 30c – Muscle pain, joint pain from an injury. Bruised and sore-to-touch pain.

Hypericum 30c – Nerve pain. Shooting lightning-like pains.

Calendula 30c – Pain on the skin from a cut or scrape. Painful wounds. Sharp pain.

Ledum – Pain from crushing injuries. Symptoms feel better from cold applications.

Symphytum 30c – Bone pain. The bone may be sore to touch.

Ruta 30c – Tendon and ligament pain. Old sprains that don't heal all the way from Arnica. Pain in the tendons is worse at night. Tendinitis.

Bryonia 30c – Any pain that is worse from motion. A joint that was injured can't be moved or the pain will return.

Rhus tox 30c – Pain with stiffness. The stiffness is worse from cold damp weather and better from a hot bath and/or continued motion. The person can feel like a rusty gate; that is, they feel stiff on beginning to move, then less stiff as they continue to move.

PANIC – SEE Fear and Anxiety

PHANTOM LIMB PAIN – SEE ALSO Nerve Injury

Hypericum 30c – Shooting pains in the area of the amputation.

Allium cepa 30c – Pain continues long after an injury. Pain feels worse from a warm room. Patient feels sleepiness in the daytime. Bloating occurrs easily in the abdomen. May have sinus condition with mucous that burns the upper lip. May have phantom limb pains.

POISON IVY –
This condition is very treatable with homeopathy.

Rhus-tox 30c – Use for itching of the skin. If this remedy does not help, then see a professional homeopath. There are many other remedies that can be tried.

POISONING – FOOD OR WATER –
For food and water related bacterial or viral ingestion.

Arsenicum (Metal album) 30c – This is the first remedy to take for any type of FOOD POISONING. For nausea, vomiting and diarrhea. This remedy has helped more people around the world with this condition than any other remedy. It often works so quickly that you will wonder if you were actually getting sick. Take it as soon as you begin to feel any nausea. Do not fear this remedy because of what it is made from, as there are no atoms of arsenic in the 30c potency. I have personally used it many times. It has a tremendous power to stimulate the immune system into killing unwanted bacteria and viruses in the stomach and intestines.

Veratrum album 30c – If the Arsenicum 30c does not help, or only helps a little, then take this remedy. The symptoms can be very severe when this remedy is indicated, i.e., the vomiting won't stop, diarrhea won't stop or there are vomiting and diarrhea at the same time. For when you *are vomiting and* feel *very cold and can't get warm.* Craving for cold drinks and sour foods. Have symptoms of a COLD NOSE and COLD FEELING ALL OVER. Also, may be feeling weakness and loss of vitality.

PUNCTURE WOUNDS –
Bites, stepping on sharp objects and hand injuries.

Tetanus is often associated with *rust,* especially rusty nails, but this concept is somewhat misleading. Objects that accumulate rust are often found outdoors, or in places that harbor anaerobic bacteria. The rust itself does not cause tetanus nor does it contain more C. tetani bacteria. The rough surface of a rusty metal merely provides a prime habitat for a C. tetani endospore to reside. The nail affords a means to puncture skin and deliver endospore into the wound. An endospore is a non-metabolizing survival structure that begins to metabolize and cause infection once in an adequate environment. Because C. tetani is an anaerobic bacterium, it and its endospores survive well in an environment that lacks *oxygen.* Hence, stepping on a nail (rusty or not) may result in a tetanus infection. The low-oxygen (anaerobic) environment is provided by the same object which causes a *puncture wound.* **This** puncture wound delivers endospores to a suitable environment for growth. Tetanus can be prevented by *vaccination* with tetanus toxoid. The Center for Disease Control (CDC) recommends that adults receive a *booster* vaccine every ten years.

It is interesting that the standard of care to prevent tetanus, that being a tetanus vaccination, uses the same principle as homeopathy. If this vaccination was tested in smaller doses, it may have the same effect with less side effects.

Ledum 30c – Useful to use if in situations such as stepping on a nail, a cat bite or mosquito bite. Use if experiencing dull achy pains.

Hypericum 30c – Useful for puncture wounds that could lead to tetanus. Useful for shooting pains. I would take a dose of Ledum 30c and a dose of Hypericum 30c for any deep puncture wound. Take them about an hour apart.

Tetaninum 30c – This is the homeopathic dilution of the tetanus bacterium. If a patient was in the process of developing tetanus, it may be of some use, as the vaccination takes at least two weeks to have an effect.

SCRAPES – SEE ALSO Skin Injuries

Use regular fist aid measures such as cleaning the wound with water.Apply pressure if there is bleeding.

Calendula cream is useful for any scrape. It will help the pain and prevent infection. If the wound is deeper, then also use:

Calendula 30c – This remedy can be taken as a liquid internally to support the healing process.

SHOCK –

Such as from a car accident or some other physical trauma.

Aconite 30c – Use when have fear from threat of death, panic feeling after a car accident or fear that death was almost realized.

Arnica 30c – Useful for soreness and bruising, pain from an injury, and/or a feeling that everything is moving in slow motion. Denial of the injury; says he is feeling well, but obviously he is not well. Can use for nightmares after an injury.

Arsenicum 30c – Useful for vomiting and/or diarrhea. May be chilly with a desire to feel warm.

SPRAINS AND STRAINS OF JOINTS –

These usually occur as the result of a sports injury.

Arnica 30c – First remedy to take for any injury. Useful for pain from trauma, a sports injury, falls, sprains, bruises and sore bruises.

Ledum 30c – Useful for sore swollen joints when relief is gained from cold applications.

Rhus tox 30c – Use for older injuries which are stiff and sore. The stiffness is worse when beginning motion and better when motion is continued. The pain is better with heat but worse with cold and damp weather.

Ruta 30c – Use for old injuries like tendinitis. Use if experiencing pain at night or when at rest and worse from overuse.

Bryonia 30c – Use when pain is worse from any motion and better when kept perfectly still.

Symphytum 30c – Use for injuries to bones, bruised bones, broken bones and black eyes.

Carbo animalis 30c – Use if experiencing weakness after lifting. Helpful if experiencing weakness of the arm, neck/back or legs following an injury. Good for pain and weakness from overuse of an injured joint.

Skin Injuries, Scrapes, Cuts, Surgical Wounds –

Calendula cream is useful for any skin injury. It will help the pain and prevent infection. If the wound is deeper, then use Calendula 30c as well.

Spider Bites – see Insect Bites

HOBO SPIDER BITE –

Euphorbium latharus 30c – These bites produce a severe burning pain. There is ulceration around the bite. Take one or two doses a day. The Hobo spider can be identified by its two antennae that protrudes from the head with bulbs at the ends. Always try to collect the spider to show your health professional.

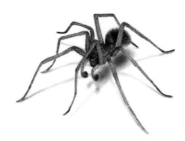

SPORTS INJURIES – SEE Injuries

Use **Arnica 30c** first. See the section on injuries.

STIFF JOINTS –

After an injury take **Arnica 30c**, then a few days later the bruising most likely will be all better. The joint may still be stiff. If Arnica is helping overall, keep taking it. If Arnica is not helping the stiffness, then consider Rhus tox or some other remedy.

Rhus tox 30c – Stiffness on beginning to move that is better from continued motion and worse from the cold damp weather.

Calcarea carbonica 30c – Stiffness that is worse from the cold damp weather. Good to take for brittle fingernails, fear of heights and/or difficulty losing weight.

Kali carbonica 30c – Stiff joints and arthritic joints. Example, he wakes up between two and three in the morning and can't sleep.

SUNBURN –
Pain from and red inflamed skin.

Cantharis 30c – For any common sunburn.

Urtica urens 30c – Hives from sunburn. Take for pain and swelling of the skin from sunburn.

SUNSTROKE, SUN HEADACHE AND SUNBURN –
Usually, there is a headache after being in the sun for too many hours.

Glonoin 30c – This is the first remedy to take for sunstroke. Take for sunstroke or a throbbing headache from becoming overheated. *Example,* after hiking in the sun all day, he experienced a pounding headache.

Belladonna 30c - Useful for any throbbing headache. *This includes eyes being very sensitive to light.*

SURGERY –
Use to prevent pain from surgery; infection from surgery; aid in the healing of surgical wounds. Listed are remedies for skin tissue healing, nerve injury and bone injury. Also, some of these remedies treat the nausea of anesthetic and anxiety before surgery.

Arnica 30c – Recommendation: Take one dose 12 to 18 hours before surgery. This can prevent excessive bleeding or bruising, reduce pain, and accelerate the overall healing process.

Calendula 30c – Recommendation: Take as soon after the surgery as possible, and then once a day for three days. This will help *prevent any infection,* reduce pain, and aid in wound healing.

Symphytum 30c – *Useful for any cutting of bone tissue,* such as dental surgery where a tooth was extracted, and the jaw bone was traumatized.

Hypericum 30c – Recommendation: Take this remedy following surgery *if a nerve was stretched or cut.* Symptoms of this include: numbness, tingling, or a sharp shooting pain.

Phosphorus 30c – Useful for excessive nausea after an anesthetic, and for a wound which won't stop bleeding.

Aconite 30c – Use for excessive anxiousness and *fear of death before surgery.* The anxiety may be accompanied by palpitations.

TAIL BONE INJURY – SEE Nerve **OR** Bone Injury
The tail bone is the last bone at the base of the spine.

Symphytum 30c – This is the first remedy to try for this condition if the tail bone is bruised.

Hypericum 30c – Take one dose of this if the nerves in the lower spine are affected. There may be shooting of pains into the buttocks or legs.

TEETHING – SEE ALSO Dental Work Remedies

TENDINITIS –
Tendons connect muscles to bones. Ligaments connect bone to bone. These remedies can be used for tendons and ligament injuries.

Ruta 30c – Useful if tendon pain is often *worse from overuse* of a joint. Repeating the same motion over and over, such as working on an assembly line or during some other structured occupation. Often, I have seen this in grocery check-out workers. Their wrists become painful from repeating the same motion over and over again. The tendons, as a result, become inflamed. Ruta will usually help when the pain is *worse at night* in the affected area. *Anxiety of conscience* is another symptom I have seen cured by this remedy. That being, they feel excessive guilt for no apparent reason. Anxiety in a closed warm room sometimes is present but not always. Useful for shoulder pains from swimming. May help eye strain or from doing the same motion over and over on an assembly line.

Symphytum 30c – This is an excellent remedy to treat any damage from overuse or trauma to connective (sinuous) tissues. The connective tissues of the body (tendons, ligaments and cartilage) have a very poor blood supply. They heal quite slowly. With this remedy, the healing is speeded up significantly. Useful when the joint feels unstable and weak. May be useful for headaches and neck pain after a whiplash to the neck. Very useful for old knee injuries. Good for weakness of the knee from overuse. May help back pain from overuse.

TENNIS ELBOW – SEE ALSO Injuries
These are the same remedies that are used for tendinitis. See above.

Ruta 30c – The pain in the elbow is worse at night. Good for sharp pains in the elbow from using it.

VOMITING AND NAUSEA – SEE ALSO Food Poisoning
The cause of any particular nausea is very specific and can range from food poisoning to motion sickness. Consult your physician. Also look under: Food Poisoning.

Bismuth 30c – Use for nausea accompanied by *severe gripping and grinding pains in the abdomen.* Example: Lies on the floor writhing in pain and has a desire for company. He has a restless angry mood but *cannot endure to be alone.* Water is vomited as soon as it touches the stomach. There is a burning feeling in the abdomen, as if a heavy load was there. The patient feels better from cold drinks.

Cocculus indicus 30c – Useful for nausea with vertigo. The symptoms are worse from the smell of food cooking. Symptoms are worse from the loss of sleep.

Ipecacuanha 30c – Useful for nausea and vomiting. The stomach feels relaxed and hangs down. The tongue is usually clean. May have nausea with bleeding. May experience nausea or vomiting with a gagging cough.

Phosphorus 30c – Helpful for nausea accompanied by a craving for ice water. Use if vomiting as soon as the water warms up in the stomach.

Tabacum 30c – For nausea when there is a desire to uncover the abdomen to cold air. Patient may have faintness with nausea and /or vomiting on the least motion. Nausea may be like sea-sickness. A cold sweat may be accompanied with the nausea. Patient may desire the open air which lessens the nausea.

WHIPLASH –
These can be mild to severe types of injuries. Consult a professional, such as a chiropractor, after a whiplash injury.

WEAKNESS –
Injuries to the spine, nerves and muscles can result in body weakness.

Carbo animalis 30c – For weakness after an injury. *Example:* A fall, sports injury, or car accident. Weeks after the injury, lifting heavy things brings on profound weakness the following day. *Example:* A month after the car accident, she still could not pick up her children. If she did, she would experience weakness and weariness in all her muscles the next day.

Wounds – see also Cuts and Scrapes

Calendula 30c – This is the remedy to take *for any wound* or after any surgery to the body. It is good for CUTS, SCRAPES and ABRASIONS to the skin. It will take some of the pain away, keep the wound free of infection, and help the wound to heal rapidly.

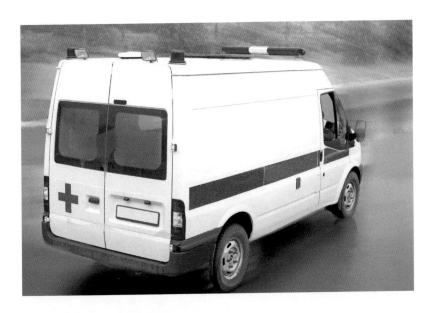

My brother Jeff has been a paramedic for over 20 years. Here is his experience with wound care:
"Clean the wound with water and mild soap, shampoo or regular hand soap. Wounds with dirt or gravel need to be scrubbed! Solutions with antimicrobials are useless because the whole point is to rinse away everything. Nobody leaves soap on their hands long enough, anyway, for the 'anti microbial' to have an effect (just another gimmick). On the ambulance, we use saline irrigation (water mixed with some salt). No soap is used because it is messy and requires too much water to rinse. Save that for

the hospital.

Inevitably, the most important point is to rinse and rinse again, and then protect from secondary infection with a dry breathable dressing. Allow the wound to dry and heal (scabbing is a defense barrier).

Also, remember wounds heal from the inside out and that a pus discharge on the wound is normal. It does not necessarily mean infection. Pus is the normal way for a body to rid itself of dead cells and other unwanted tissue; thus, not over taxing the lymphatics. As you know, redness and abnormal swelling with increasing pain are signs of infection. Small infections to any wound are normal; signs of infection should not be worsening after 36-48 hours."
– *Jeff Olsen - Paramedic Chief - Station 408 Grand Forks.*

CHAPTER 3

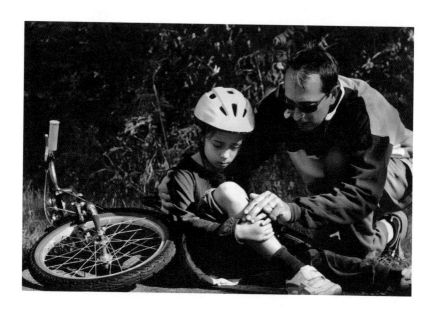

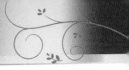

Research

How effective is homeopathy in treating certain ailments? How does it work when used in such a small dose? Can it be used for epidemics? What is its scientific basis?

I have collected many studies and posted them on my web site:
http://snohomishwellness.com/research-and-homeopathy

Some helpful definitions before you continue:

- **Double-blind:** a study in which neither the researcher nor the participant know if either a placebo or a drug were given

- **Placebo:** a sugar pill or similar non-drug substance with the appearance of the real drug.

- **Placebo-controlled:** a study with two groups, one given a placebo and the other the drug.

- **Randomized:** the participants in the study are placed in either group randomly to create a more equal mix of traits and factors between groups.

Studies can be found on the following websites:
http://www.facultyofhomeopathy.org/research
https://www.hri-research.org
http://www.homeopathycenter.org/research
http://www.homeopathyeurope.org/Research
http://www.audesapere.in
www.marlev.com/Articles/PositiveHomeopathy.pdf
http://hpathy.com/scientific-research/database-of-positive-homeopathy-research-studies

Here is an example:

The Lancet published the most significant and comprehensive review of homeopathic research ever published in its September 20, 1997, issue. This article was a meta-analysis of 89 blinded, randomized, placebo-controlled clinical trials. The authors conclude that the clinical effects of homeopathic medicines are not simply the results of placebo.

The researchers uncovered 186 studies, of which 119 were double-blind and/or randomized placebo-control trials and 89 of these met pre-defined criteria for inclusion into a pooled meta-analysis. The researchers found that by pooling the 89 trials together, homeopathic medicines had more than 2 times greater (2.45) effect than the placebo.

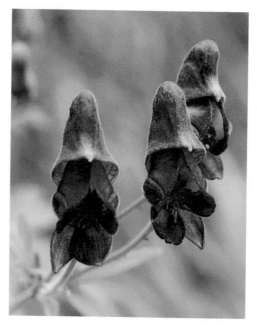

Aconite Plant

GLOSSARY

Acute illness – Usually a self-limiting illness. There is a gradual onset of symptoms followed by a crisis, which can end in resolution, or in extreme cases, in death. The flu is an example of an acute illness.

Allopathic – Regular medicine, where large doses are used to treat illness. The term coined by Samuel Hahnemann to differentiate homeopathic practices from conventional medicine, based on the types of treatments used. When used by homeopaths, the term 'allopathy' has always referred to a principle of administering substances that produce the opposite effect of the disease. *Examples:* Aspirin to treat pain, antibiotics to treat infections, cortisone to treat inflammation.

Antidote – A substance that will nullify the effect of a homeopathic remedy when exposed to the recipient patient. Coffee, camphor, essential oils and strong chemicals are the most common antidotes.

Botanica tincture – The concentration used in the preparation of herbal medicines. One part of a finely chopped herb is added to ten parts of 30% alcohol. It is shaken every day for two weeks, then strained and corked in a dark glass bottle. Mixtures of alcohol and water dissolve nearly all of the relevant ingredients of an herb, and at the same time, act as a preservative. This is also called a 'mother tincture'. Botanical tinctures are the first step in making homeopathic dilutions.

Conditions Homeopathy Can Treat – Some of the conditions which homeopathy treats include: abdominal complaints, allergies, anxiety, depression, arthritis, back injuries, behavior and learning disorders, the effects of car accidents, chronic fatigue, depression, ear infections, eating disorders, eczema, fibromyalgia, flu, food poisoning, grief, gynecological problems, hay fever, headaches, hormonal imbalances, infectious diseases, insomnia, physical trauma, psoriasis, sinusitis, sports injuries, sunstroke, urinary tract infections, wound care, and various other first aid, acute and chronic conditions.

Chronic illness – A lengthy continued illness, usually present for six months or longer. There can be exacerbations or a worsening of symptoms during the illness. For example, asthma is usually a chronic illness. At times it is worse, depending on many factors.

Combination remedy – Two or more individual homeopathic remedies mixed together in one container. This is a less ideal method than giving one medicine at a time. Practiced too often, it can produce side effects, antidote (make ineffective) the correct medicine, and confuse the symptoms. This will prevent the practitioner from finding the true simillimum (see definition below).

Diagnosis – Homeopathic diagnosis is the process of determining the medicine that is needed. This is accomplished by undertaking a lengthy interview to identify the history, signs and symptoms of the patient. By means of the interview process, a person's symptoms are identified in as much detail as possible.

Healing system – That part of any living organism which generates defensive reactions to adverse stimuli. It guides or controls the natural, innate, healing process. This is known in biology as the 'mechanisms of homeostasis' or defense mechanism.

Health – definition of – The ability to think logically and coherently, with clarity, rationality, flexibility and creativity. Health creates a sense of purpose; a definite sense of individual identity. To be free of pain and physical limitations. To be able to use ones full potential.

Homeopathic dose – One dose consists of five to eight granules of a particular remedy or one teaspoon of a liquid remedy. The actual amount of substance is not the main factor in the definition of one homeopathic dose. There is some variation in the amounts taken. For example, there would be little difference between taking ten or five granules. One tablespoon or one teaspoon of the liquid would not make any difference to the effective dose. In contrast to the amount taken at one time, the strength of the remedy makes a very large difference to the effect of the remedy. A 6c is weaker than a 12c, and a 30c is still stronger; therefore, can be taken less often. The 200c is stronger. This is not recommended for home use unless it is clear the 30c has acted well but has not been able to cure the last 10 to 35 percent of the illness. If any remedy is repeated too often, it can produce unwanted side effects. Repeat the remedy only when there has been a plateau of symptom relief or when the symptoms start to return.

Homeopathic proving – A proving is the method of determining the healing properties of an individual remedy. Healthy people are given diluted doses of a particular medicine. The temporary symptoms which are produced are carefully recorded. For example, the proving symptoms of 'onion' are burning watery eyes. If a homeopathic dilution of onion (Allium cepa) was given to a person with allergies who also had burning eyes, then a cure could result. (As long as all the other symptoms of the patient were also a match with the symptoms which 'onion' could create.)

Homeopathic remedy – A medicine or remedy, is that substance which, through provings on healthy people and from clinical experience, is known to produce a similar symptom picture to that experienced by the patient. A remedy is homeopathic, not only by virtue of its method of preparation, dilution

/succussion, but also by virtue of its ability to produce a similar symptom picture. Combination medicines, mixtures of various remedies in one bottle, are not homeopathic. As such, a combination remedy has never been tested to determine what range of symptoms it will cure.

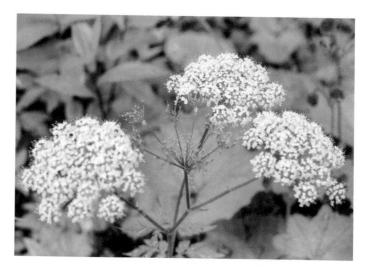

Eupatorium Perfoliatum

Healing Steps – what happens when a remedy is taken - Diagram A, below, illustrates a healthy, strong healing mechanism. The four large arrows represent the strength of both the individual cells and the strength of the body as a whole.

An individual with this level of health will be able to resist many insults of stress and not become sick. For example, they may be exposed to a strep bacterial infection, and the bacteria may live in their throat for some time, but no symptoms will result.[1]

Although this is a simplistic diagram, it communicates the idea the healing system of the body is intelligent, reactive, and if the body can, it will always cure the illness on the mental level first,

---

1   This has been confirmed by lab tests done on people with no symptoms, but, in fact, they still carry the pathogenic bacteria. Also, it has been found that some people become very sick from bacteria that, for most of us, are benign and usually do not cause any illness.

then the emotional level, and finally the physical level last of all.

Diagram A

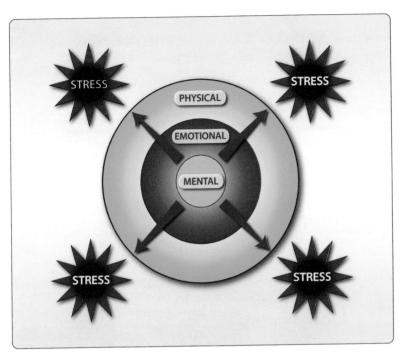

There are very few people in our society with this level of overall health. Most of us inherit a susceptibility to at least one illness and/or have a major stress in life that creates a new susceptibility.

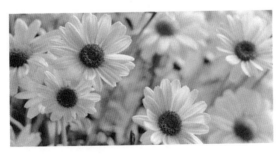

Chamomilla Plant

Slightly susceptible defense mechanism –

Diagram B, below, illustrates the conditions of a minor susceptibility. In this situation, a stressor can 'trigger' the susceptibility, and some symptoms can arise. An acute illness or an injury that is slow to heal are examples.

Diagram B

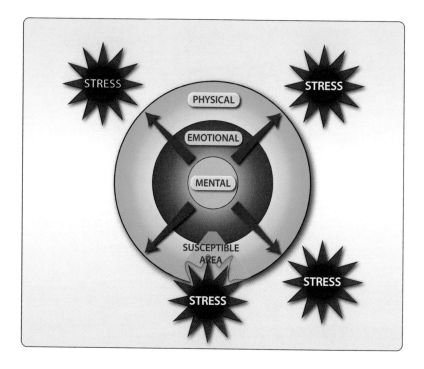

In this next example - Diagram C, there is a moderate susceptibility combined with a long-continued stress allowing for a chronic illness or very severe acute illness to arise. This could, for example, be mild arthritis, one or two moderate headaches a month, easily triggered irritability, anxiety or sadness.

Diagram C

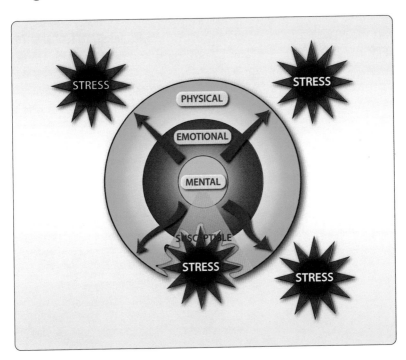

The list of moderate symptom combinations is endless. There are millions of people who live productive lives while enduring a depleted level of health of this severity. In a sense, this is the norm of our society, but it does not have to be endured. If we commit ourselves to the value of treating the cause of symptoms, rather than suppressing them, then this typical state of illness will not have to continue.

Severely susceptible defense mechanism -
Diagram D below shows the healing systems of the body in disarray.

Diagram D

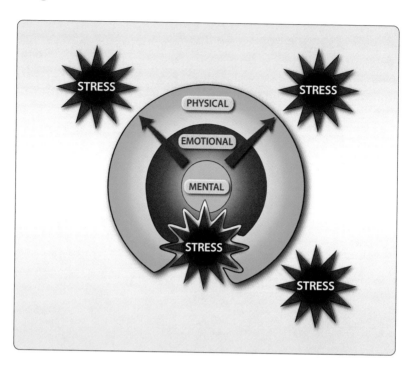

A person with this level of health would suffer from continuous chronic physical symptoms, severe depression or anxiety or some other mental condition. These symptoms would be influenced to a great extent by the genetic inheritance of that person's family. Even a minor stress will, with the susceptibility depicted above, produce the most severe types of acute and chronic illnesses. Some of these cases are not curable with homeopathy, and only the palliation of symptoms can be achieved or an increase in overall health, but not a return to complete health. This depends on many factors. If the person is young, they only need one to three remedies, then the prognosis is much better, and a lot more can be achieved.

THE EFFECTS OF HOMEOPATHIC MEDICINE ON THE DEFENSE MECHANISM –

If the correct homeopathic medicine is given, and it matches the overall individuality of the patient's susceptibility by more than 95 percent, we call this the simillimum. If the match is less accurate, then only a few symptoms, or none at all, will diminish. The simillimum has the potential to permanently rebuild the systems of homeostasis.

Diagram E, below, shows the initial action of the homeopathic medicine. It presses up against the already weakened areas of the defense mechanism. During this stage, the healing system of the body 'perceives' the remedy. This is the primary action of the remedy, and for a brief time (usually one day in the case of a chronic illness) the symptoms can be made temporarily worse. For first aid and acute illness, we do not notice this aggravation of symptoms.

Diagram E

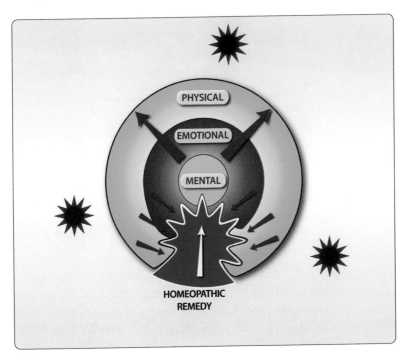

FINAL STAGE OF HEALING

In the next stage, shown in Diagram F, below, the healing system evaluates the effects of the homeopathic medicine.

Diagram F

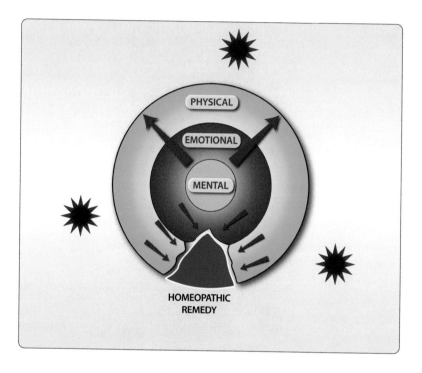

As the defense mechanism is now focused on the area that needs to be cured first, it gathers its resources for a reaction that over-comes the initial effect of the remedy and, in turn, overcomes the disease process.

This is the secondary action of the remedy. In this final stage, the healing system produces a reaction/strategy that is intelligent and strong enough to overcome the effect of the homeopathic medicine and now begins to react to the illness in a curative way.

Real healing now occurs, and the person will feel the effects of this active process within a short time – usually within minutes to hours in a first aid situation, a day for an acute illness, and about a week for an illness with chronic symptoms.

Once the healing process has achieved its objective, the symptoms of the illness gradually diminish. The healing systems of the body now have the renewed ability to maintain health at a stronger and more integrated level of homeostasis. The susceptibility is 'cured'; thus, stress no longer has a place to gain a foothold to begin a disease process.

Below in diagram G, the continuation of the healing process is shown.

Diagram G

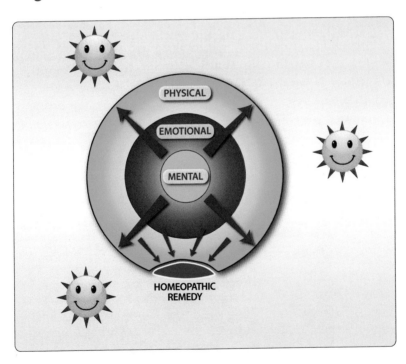

When a homeopathic medicine has been taken, which has the exact similarity to the patient's illness, and which results in an overall improvement in health, it is called the 'simillimum,' 'constitutional' or 'classical' homeopathic remedy. The remedy has brought about a permanent overall improvement in the patient's health. One medicine was used at a time, and the minimum dilution was used to bring about this new level of health. Notice how a person with regained health can now perceive stress as a positive challenge.

The underlying causes of the illness are; therefore, cured.

Although the diagrams above give us an intuitive understanding of how the remedy works, it is not a complete scientific explanation. First of all, the remedy is not understood yet in terms of an exact force or exact particle we can measure. Also, what is the receptor that it interacts with on the cellular level? We do not know this. Further, we do not know the exact mechanism of the healing system itself in any kind of concrete way as we do, for example, know how a car engine works. It would be academically interesting to know all of this. It would lead to a complete application of homeopathy into all the areas of medicine that could benefit from it and applications that we have not even considered. For example, animals and plants also possess a healing system that, when compromised, need a diagnosis and treatment. For a complete explanation, see *The New Science of Homeopathy*, by Steve Olsen.

Having said that, we still can use each remedy safely and experience its healing effects.

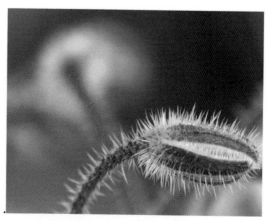

Symphytum [Cumfrey plant]

Summary:

The cause of a disease is ultimately determined by the susceptibility of the person's healing system combined with an external stressor, such as bacteria, viruses, physical trauma, toxic substance or emotional stress.

The factor of susceptibility is usually left out when a medical condition is explained by the media. *Example:* "There is a new strain of the flu virus causing pneumonia." If that was true, then everyone who was exposed to this virus would get pneumonia, but we know that is not true. Only those people who have a susceptibility to pneumonia can get it from a particular virus. For example, the bacteria that 'causes' strep throat was found in about 20% of people who did not even have a sore throat. This concept is well known in medicine; one can be a carrier of a bacteria or virus but not have any symptoms. Why? It is because those people are not susceptible to it.

The health of the defense mechanism is inherited, then influenced through life by various stressful or positive effects upon it. There are two steps by which the healing system of the body produces a cure in response to a homeopathic medicine.

Step one: The medicine interacts with a receptor of some kind producing a temporary aggravation of the symptoms. This is the primary action of the medicine.

Step two: The body reacts in the opposite way to resist against this influence. This healing response is the secondary action, which restores normal health to the body.

The outcome of an illness is dependent upon the ability of a sick person to cure him/herself. This is determined primarily by the accuracy of the homeopathic medicine given, and the relative strength of the person's healing systems.

Homeostasis – medical definition - The tendency of a system, especially the physiological system, to maintain internal stability, owing to the coordinated response of its parts to any situation or stimulus tending to disturb its normal condition or function.

The tendency of an organism or cell to regulate its internal conditions, such as the pH chemical composition of its body fluids, so as to maintain health and functioning, regardless of outside conditions. The organism or cell maintains homeostasis by monitoring its internal conditions and responding appropriately when these conditions deviate from their optimal state. The maintenance of a steady body temperature in warm-blooded animals is an example of homeostasis. In human beings, the homeostatic regulation of body temperature involves such mechanisms as sweating when the internal temperature becomes excessive and shivering to produce heat, as well as the generation of heat through metabolic processes when the internal temperature falls too low.

Diseases that result from a homeostatic imbalance include diabetes, dehydration, infections, diseases caused by a toxin present in the bloodstream, arthritis, headaches. Almost any illness is partly the result of a weakness or deficit in homeostasis. So every illness, almost, can benefit from a stronger reaction in homeostasis. From a textbook of regular medicine, we find this quote:

"Just as we live in a constantly changing world, so do the cells and tissues survive in a constantly changing microenvironment. The 'normal' or 'physiologic' state then is achieved by adaptive responses to the ebb and flow of various stimuli permitting the cells and tissues to adapt and to live in harmony within their microenvironment. Thus, homeostasis is preserved. It is only when the stimuli become more severe, or the response of the organism breaks down, that disease results - a generalization as true for the whole organism as it is for the individual cell."[2]

Originally, in the homeopathic literature, this idea of homeostasis or self-healing, was defined as being the result of a "vital force." In modern literature this term is no longer in use, instead, the term homeostasis is used to define the same idea.

Here is what Hahnemann said and we can see that the meaning is the same.

"When a man (or woman) falls ill, it is, at first, only this self-sustaining vital principle everywhere present in the organism (homeostasis) which is untuned (out of balance) by the dynamic influence of the hostile disease agent upon it. It is only this vital principle, thus untuned, which brings about in the organism the disagreeable sensations and abnormal functions that we call disease. Being invisible, and recognizable solely by its effects on the organism, it can express itself and reveal its 'untune'-ment only by pathological manifestations in feeling and functions as disease symptom."
   ~ The Organon of Medicine by Samuel Hahnemann.

Characteristics of Homeostasis: It can act on the molecular level, cellular level, organ level and systems level, and/or usually inter-related on all of these levels. Homeostasis, for example, can act to repair DNA chromosomes. An extreme example of this can be found in bacterium Deinococcus radiodurans [see below].

Homeostasis is, therefore, that part of the living organism

---

2   (Pathologic Basis of Disease, third edition, S.L. Robbins MD, R.S. Cotran MD, V.K. Kumar MD. 1984, W.P. Saunders Company)

which initiates and coordinates the healing processes. All living systems have a relative resistance to toxicity. Homeostasis can work to repair DNA. All the biological and molecular steps of homeostasis are yet to be defined, but we know, at least, that the cells have receptors, and so this system is not as invisible as it was in Hahnemann's time.

Generally, homeostasis can be achieved with proper nutrition, exercise, healthy lifestyle, and a positive emotional environment. If these are maintained and the person is still sick, then one has to look for the maintaining cause of the illness (genetic and epigenetic susceptibility; predisposing factors). It has been found that a homeopathic medicine can affect the epigenome to bring it back to a healthier state.

How do medicines (drugs) affect homeostasis, and how is this achieved? Some of the best work being done on this subject is in the field of hormesis.

Extreme example of homeostasis -

Meet the Super-bug; by John Travis; If a massive nuclear war ever blanketed the planet with radioactive fallout, cockroaches, despite all the jokes, we would be goners. A bacterium known as Deinococcus radiodurans might survive, however. Its name, which means "strange berry that withstands radiation," indicates the reason that the microbe fascinates scientists. Labeled the world's toughest bacterium by The Guinness Book of World Records, D. radiodurans shrugs off doses of radiation many thousands of times stronger than those that would kill a person.

Scientists have also established that the microbe doesn't simply shield its DNA from the radiation. It, instead, has an unprecedented ability to repair genetic damage.

Scientists usually measure radiation in units called rads, and a dose of 500 to 1000 rads is lethal to the average person. In contrast, depending upon conditions for its growth, D. radiodurans thrives after exposures of up to 1.5 million rads. Cool or freeze the microbe, and it may survive 3.0 million rads.

Bacteria that form hard capsules called spores can withstand
large amounts of radiation but not as much as can D. radiodurans,
which doesn't form a spore. "It is supreme in its radiation resistance," says Michael J. Daly of the Uniformed Services University
of the Health Sciences in Bethesda, Md.

Working with his colleague Kenneth W. Minton, Daly has for
many years sought to explain how the bacterium's DNA-repair
system accounts for its exceptional hardiness. "I was interested
in DNA repair, so why not study it in an organism that does it
better than anything else?" he asks.

Indeed, D. radiodurans faces quite a challenge when it is hit
with millions of rads. Literally shattering the bacterium's genetic
material into hundreds of fragments, the radiation creates
complete breaks in the microbe's double-stranded molecules of
DNA.

A double-strand break is the most difficult kind of DNA damage
to repair. The well-studied bacterium Escherichia coli, for example,
usually can't survive more than two or three double-strand
breaks. Yet within a few hours, D. radiodurans begins to stitch its
thoroughly fractured DNA together, and it eventually resurrects
a genome free of mutations.

"There are no natural environments that have fluxes of radiation
that could have selected for this organism," says Daly.

A few years ago, Battista's group tested an alternative hypothesis. Noting that D. radiodurans can also withstand extended
periods without water. Robert G. Murray of the University of
Western Ontario in London, Ontario, many years ago put forth
the theory that its DNA-repair system evolved to combat desic-
cation. A much more common problem for bacteria, dehydration
helps explain the popularity of spores: The capsules hold in the
last available drops of water.

While the evolutionary origin of D. radiodurans' repair system remains unresolved, so does the system's secret to success. Daly and Minton have studied two DNA-repair strategies employed by the bacterium.

Initially, it uses a process called single-strand annealing to reconnect some chromosome fragments. Its more crucial method, known as homologous recombination, uses a protein called RecA to patch double-strand breaks. After searching through the multiple copies of the genome that exist in each bacterium, RecA and associated proteins identify an intact copy of a DNA sequence that needs repair and uses that copy to mend and rejoin the broken strand.

"Yet neither single-strand annealing nor homologous recombination is unique to D. radiodurans. "Those systems alone can't account for its radiation resistance," says Daly.

Nor does redundancy in the microbe's genome explain the phenomenon. Four to 10 copies of the D. radiodurans genome exist in each bacterium. These backup copies are crucial because they increase the odds that a mutated gene will have an undamaged counterpart. Battista's group has shown that when D. radiodurans grows under conditions that reduce its number of genome copies, the bacterium becomes more vulnerable to radiation. Nevertheless, other bacteria also keep extra copies of their genome.

"The fact that there are multiple copies of the genome is not in and of itself a sufficient explanation for why they're so radiation resistant. They have to have the capacity to use that redundant genetic information in a way that most organisms cannot," says Battista.

Daly and Minton have proposed that, to speed homologous recombination, the bacterium aligns copies of its genome so that identical DNA sequences are near each other. Since bacterial chromosomes usually come in circles, this theory invokes pictures of stacked loops of DNA, resembling a roll of hard candies, and so has earned the name the Life Saver hypothesis. Battista finds this concept attractive and even has microscope images of the microbe's chromosomes that suggest there's some unusual organization among them. "The hypothesis is probably going to hold up. The Life Savers are there. We've got really pretty pictures," he says.

Battista also notes that when he irradiates normal strains of D. radiodurans, the Life Saver arrangement remains. Yet, when he zaps mutant strains that can't repair DNA, the Life Savers vanish.

In this case, as with the other genomes, scientists have pinned down the roles of only about two-thirds of the genes.[3]

Materia Medica - A text describing the medicines that are used in the practice of homeopathy. Each medicine is described according to the symptoms it is known to be able to cure.

Organon – Abbreviation for The Organon of Medicine. The text which lays down Hahnemann's foundation of homeopathic theory and practice. The first edition was published in 1810. The sixth and last edition was probably completed in 1842, the year in which Hahnemann died. It was not published until 1921.

Pathology – A state of illness or disease which is marked by changes, imbalances to normal function, (physiology, biochemistry), body structure or states of wellness. Pathology does not always produce symptoms that can be felt. For example, high blood pressure is a pathology, but it is "silent'" and has no sensation associated with it. A tumor in the bowel is also a pathology that usually has no symptoms in its early stages.

---

3   From Science News, Vol. 154, No. 24, December 12, 1998, p. 376. Copyright ©1998 by Science Service.
References: Lange, C.C., L.P. Wackett, K.W. Minton, and M.J. Daly. 1998. Engineering a recombinant Deinococcus radiodurans for organopollutant degradation in radioactive mixed waste environments. Nature Biotechnology 16(October).

Polycrest – A fully tested (proven) and commonly used homeopathic medicine which is useful for a wide variety of ailments and diseases. Sulphur, Phosphorus, and Lycopodium are examples of homeopathic remedies which are considered to be polycrests.

Potency – The strength or power of a remedy. The potency increases as the concentration decreases, provided that there is vigorous mixing – succussion – at each step of the dilution process. 6x is weaker than 6c. Then 30x and 30c, then 200x and 200c are the strongest.

Potentization – The pharmacological process of creating a homeopathic medicine by means of a process of dilution with distilled water and subsequent succussion of each dilution. The chemistry and physics of this process is not fully understood, as one normally would find less of a reaction with a more dilute solution.

Repertory – An index of symptoms (called rubrics) with corresponding remedies. Each rubric contains a list of remedies which are known to have cured that symptom or to have demonstrated its part in a remedy proving. For example the rubric: Ear Pain contains the remedies: Aconite, Belladonna, Phosphorus, and Sulphur.

Simillimum – The one remedy whose symptoms are most similar to the totality of the symptoms of the patient. The simillimum will bring about the most gentle, rapid and permanent cure of a particular patient's symptoms. A medicine that is close, but not the true simillimum, will sometimes have partial effects, then a relapse may occur.

Succussion – The physical shaking of the remedy dilution in order to create a 'kinetic' effect. Before taking a homeopathic remedy, one should shake it very well. In experiments on homeopathic medicines, when there was no succussion process, then the remedy seemed to lose its therapeutic effect.

Susceptibility – The susceptibility to illness is inherited from our parents, and then further affected by what we eat, medical drugs taken, our lifestyle and the emotional experiences of childhood. If the susceptibility of inheritance is mild, then with a very positive lifestyle, the illnesses we develop will also be mild. If though, there are severe emotional shocks or traumas to which we can not recover from, then a new layer of susceptibility develops and this in turn leads to the beginning of a new chronic illness. The suppression of isolated symptoms of an acute illness or chronic illness can also create new layers of susceptibility, leading to a new chronic illness or worsening of the original one.

Symptoms – A stress interacting with a specific susceptibility produces sensations of illness or signs of illness called symptoms. The symptoms are the language of the defense mechanism in the sense that they tell us where the defense system is broken or injured. They can be sensations that one feels, such as pain, objective findings, such as swelling or emotions such as depression.

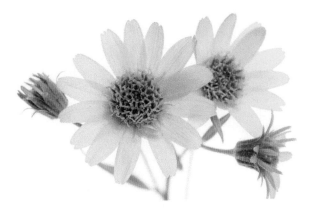

Arnica Montana

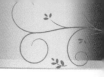

It is not sufficient to read this review and expect to be proficient at Cardio Pulmonary Resuscitation (CPR). There are many courses available in most communities, often offered by the local fire department, ambulance station or hospital.

The first step in all CPR is to activate the 911 Emergency Medical Response system. Identify a bystander by name or by pointing to them to do this for you. Make sure they understand and agree. If you are alone, call 911 and then begin first aid. To help you administer effective first aid instantaneously, follow these steps:

Open the airway and check for breathing –
Gently tilt the head back and check for breathing by putting your cheek near the person's mouth. Look for chest movement and listen for sounds of breathing.

Remove any obvious obstruction –
Place your thumb inside the mouth to hold down the tongue, then sweep index finger inside mouth if an obstruction is seen.

Check for a pulse –
Use the first two fingers of your hand, not your thumb. The surest place to feel for a pulse is on the front of the neck, next to the throat.

If there is no pulse, this means the heart has stopped and you will need to do chest compressions along with rescue breathing. If there is a pulse but no breathing, then only do the rescue breathing.

Rescue breathing
Adult (2 breaths) –
Pinch the nose closed. Take a full breath and place your lips around the person's lips to make a good seal. Blow into the mouth until the chest rises. This will take 2 seconds for a full

inflation. Raise your head and allow the person's chest to fall. Repeat.

Child/baby (5 breaths) – Seal your lips tightly around both the mouth and nose for a baby, or pinch the nose and seal your lips around just the mouth for a child. Blow into the mouth until the chest rises. Give 5 breaths in a row, being sure to let the chest fall each time.

Assess for circulation –
Check for signs of circulation: normal breathing, coughing or movement. If YES, continue Rescue breathing (step 3 above). If NO, continue to step 5.

Begin CPR - Adult –
Lean over the person with your arms straight and elbows locked. Place one of your palms on top of the other hand. Place the heel of your bottom hand on the center of the breastbone. Press down vertically on the breastbone by flexing your body at the hips, depressing the person's chest by 1½ - 2 inches. Alternate 15 chest compressions with 2 breaths of rescue breathing.

Child aged 1-7 –
Position the heel of only one of your hands on the center of the child's breastbone. Press down firmly 1-1½ inches. Alternate 5 chest compressions with 1 rescue breath. If over 8, give adult treatment.

Baby – Place the tips of two of your fingers in the center of the baby's breastbone. Press down firmly ½ -1 inch. Alternate 5 chest compressions with 1 rescue breath.

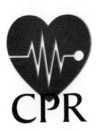

SUGGESTED READING

On-Line Courses –
http://snohomishwellness.com/similia-study-group

Homeopathic Theory –
Hahnemann, Samuel. **Organon of Medicine.** 6th Edition.

Vithoulkas, George. **The Science of Homeopathy.**

Kent, James. T. **Lectures on Homeopathic Philosophy.**

Materia Medicas –
Boericke, William. **Pocket Manual of Homeopathic Materia Medica.**

Kent, James. T. **Lectures on Homeopathic Materia Medica.** Reprint.

Nash, EB. **Leaders in Homeopathic Therapeutics.**

Allen, H.C. Allen's **Keynotes with Nosodes.**

Science of Homeopathy
Positive Drug Action, Dr. Steve Olsen

Repertory, a book to look up individual symptoms and the remedies that have been known to treat those symptoms.

Schroyens, Frederik, ed. Synthethis: Repertorium Homeopathicum Syntheticum.
These and other homeopathic books can be ordered from:

Homeopathic Educational Services: 1-800-359-9051
2036 Blake St. Berkeley, CA 94704
mail@homeopathic.com or www.homeopathic.com

Pharmacy for purchasing individual remedies - Many of the remedies suggested in this book can be purchased from a health food store, or Boiron pharmacy carries all of the remedies 1-800-blu-tube. It is suggested you order four to six remedies at a time. Order in liquid 15 ml, 30ml or multi-dose tube of solid granules.

Suggested contents of a first aid remedy kit:
Arnica montana 30c – multi-dose tube Arnica cream 20 grams
Arsenicum album 30c, multi-dose tube
Veratrum album 30c, multi-dose tube
Calendula Officinalis 30c, multi-dose tube
Calendula cream 20 grams. – the second most used remedy
Hypericum Perforatum 30c, multi-dose tube
Symphytum officinalis 30c, multi-dose tube
Ledum Pulustre 30c, multi-dose tube.
Ruta Graveolens 30c, multi-dose tube.
Rhus Toxicodendron 30c, multi-dose tube
Bryonia Alba 30c, multi-dose tube
Carbo Animalis 30c, multi-dose tube
Apis Mellifica 30c, multi-dose tube
Ignatia Amara 30c, multi-dose tube
Aconite Napellus 30c, multi-dose tube.
Cantharis 30c, multi-dose tube.
Glonoin 30c, multi-dose tube.
Belladonna 30c, multi-dose tube.
Cocculus indicus 30c, multi-dose tube.
Tabacum 30c, multi-dose tube.
Phosphorus 30c, multi-dose tube

Journal and Professional Organizations

National Center for Homeopathy
801 North Fairfax Street
Suite 306 Alexandria, VA 22314
Ph. 1- (877) 624-0613 or 1- (703) 548-7790
http://NationalCenterforHomeopathy.org

Professional Organizations

The Homeopathic Academy of Naturopathic Physicians
(HANP) http://www.hanp.net

The Homeopathic Academy of Naturopathic Physicians (HANP)
is a specialty society within the profession of naturopathic
medicine, and is affiliated with the American Association of
Naturopathic Physicians.

Our purpose is to further excellence and success in the practice
of homeopathy by naturopathic physicians and provide a vehicle
for outreach into both the naturopathic and homeopathic
communities.

HANP activities include: Encouraging the development and
improvement of homeopathic curriculum at naturopathic colleges. Publishing the bi-annual journal of homeopathic practice,
Simillimum. Hosting case conferences. Offering homeopathic
continuing education seminars. Working with the homeopathic community on issues of common interest. Offering board
certification in classical homeopathy to qualified naturopathic
physicians.

American Association of Homeopathic Pharmacists (AAHP)
5112 Wilshire Dr, Santa Rosa, CA 95404
Ph. (800) 478-0421, fax. (800) 478-0421
Web: www.homeopathyresource.org

The AAHP is an association of homeopathic manufacturers,
pharmacists and others organized to serve the homeopathic
community. They are dedicated to promoting excellence in the
practice of homeopathic pharmacy, manufacturing, marketing
and distribution by supporting the requirements, criteria and
published guidelines in the HPRS, CFR, CPG as well as other
industry regulations/compendia, aimed at providing safe effective
homeopathic medicine to consumers, retailers and healthcare
practitioners.

Academy of Veterinary Homeopathy (AVH)
PO Box 9280, Wilmington, DE 19809
Ph. (866) 652-1590, fax. (866) 652-1590
Web: www.theavh.org
E-mail: office@theavh.org

The Academy of Veterinary Homeopathy establishes standards for the practice of veterinary homeopathy and advances veterinary homeopathy through education and research. Membership is open to licensed veterinarians and veterinary students in AVMA-accredited veterinary schools.

Homeopathic Pharmacopoeia Convention of the United States (HPCUS)
PO Box 2221, Southeastern, PA 19399-2221
Fax. (610) 783-5180
Web: www.hpus.com

The Homeopathic Pharmacopoeia Convention of The United States (HPCUS) publishes the Homeopathic Pharmacopoeia of the United States (HPUS). It investigates substances for inclusion, sets standards for identification, testing, and preparation of homeopathic remedies. The HPUS is recognized in the Food and Drug Act as the source of regulation of homeopathic drugs in the USA. A 501(c)(3) organization. See www.hpus.com for more information.

American Board of Homeotherapeutics (ABHt)
10418 Whitehead St, Fairfax, VA 22030
Ph. (703) 273-5250
Web: www.homeopathyusa.org/specialty-board.html

The ABHt (est. 1959), the oldest US national licensed medical professional certifying board, grants a Diplomate (advanced specialty, DHt) to a successful MD or DO candidate of its rigorous 3-part examination. A Primary Care Certificate is granted to successful Advance Practice Nurse, Physician Assistant, and MD candidates of the Primary Care Examination.

American Institute of Homeopathy (AIH)
801 N Fairfax St Ste 306, Alexandria, VA 22314-1757
Ph. (888) 445-9988, fax. (888) 445-9988
Web: www.homeopathyusa.org
E-mail: aih@homeopathyusa.org

Established in 1844, the American Institute of Homeopathy is the oldest national US medical organization. Its members are licensed medical and osteopathic physicians, dentists, advanced practice nurses, and physician assistants who practice homeopathy. The AIH strives to promote the public acceptance of homeopathy while safeguarding the interests of the profession.

Council for Homeopathic Certification (CHC)
PMB 187, 16915 SE 272nd St Ste 100, Covington, WA 98042
Ph. (866) 242-3399 (toll free in US & Canada), fax. (815) 366-7622
Web: www.homeopathicdirectory.com

The CHC has established the largest professional certification standard in North America and is open to all professional homeopaths, including both licensed and non-licensed practitioners. The CHC serves to unite the homeopathic profession under a commonly agreed level of homeopathic competence and offers the public a clear choice in finding qualified professional homeopaths.

Council on Naturopathic Medical Education
P.O. Box 178 Great Barrington, MA 01230
Ph. (413) 528-8877, Fax. (413) 528-8880
Email: staff@cnme.org

The Council on Naturopathic Medical Education's mission is quality assurance: serving the public by accrediting naturopathic medical education programs that voluntarily seek recognition that they meet or exceed CNME's standards. Students and graduates of programs accredited or preaccredited (candidacy) by CNME are eligible to apply for the naturopathic licensing examinations administered by the North American Board of Naturopathic Examiners (NABNE), and are generally eligible for state and provincial licensure in the U.S. and Canada.

Founded in 1978, CNME is accepted as the programmatic accrediting agency for naturopathic medical education by the four-year naturopathic colleges and programs in the United States and Canada, by the American and Canadian national naturopathic professional associations, and by NABNE. CNME advocates for high standards in naturopathic education, and its grant of accreditation to a program indicates prospective students and the public may have confidence in the educational quality of the program. The U.S. Secretary of Education recognizes CNME as the national accrediting agency for programs leading to the Doctor of Naturopathic Medicine (N.D. or N.M.D.) or Doctor of Naturopathy (N.D.) degree. CNME also approves postdoctoral programs (i.e., residency programs) in naturopathic medicine. Among these programs are naturopathic residencies that provide licensed naturopathic physicians with postgraduate training in naturopathic family care and other specialties. The Handbook on CNME Postdoctoral Naturopathic Medical Education (PNME) Sponsor Recognition Process and Standards contains CNME's standards for residency programs.

CNME is a member of the Association of Specialized and Professional Accreditors (ASPA) and abides by ASPA's Code of Good Practice. CNME is also a member of the Association of Accrediting Agencies of Canada.

Naturopathic Colleges:

Boucher Institute of Naturopathic Medicine 300-435 Columbia Street New Westminster, BC V3L 5N8 Canada Email: info@binm.org

Bastyr University
14500 Juanita Dr. NE
Kenmore, WA 98028-4966

Southwest College of Naturopathic Medicine & Health Sciences
2140 E. Broadway Rd. Tempe, AZ 86043

Canadian College of Naturopathic Medicine
1255 Sheppard Ave. E,
North York, ON M2K 1E2 Canada

University of Bridgeport College of Naturopathic Medicine
60 Lafayette St. Bridgeport, CT 06604

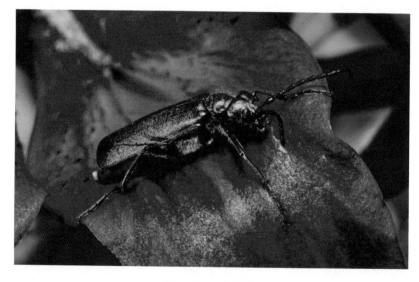

Cantharis Beetle

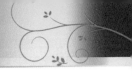

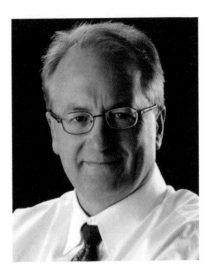

Dr. Steven Olsen – ND, DHANP

My great grandmother was a nurse in London during the 1890's, a time when Tuberculosis was prevalent. Two of her children died of TB and one survived who was later to become my grandmother. She had an extraordinary ability to listen to others and was very compassionate.

If one can listen well enough, one can perceive what needs to be cured in the patient.

My grandfather was a farmer. He was holistic in that he studied how all the resources and the natural order of things affected each other on the farm. When we get sick, the same principle applies - one factor can affect our health in different ways depending on many other factors. It is a dynamic system, but we still need to see the big picture even though it is often very complex and individualized.

My mother was a kindergarten teacher and now has a school to teach early childhood education. I think we share the appreciation of human development. Human development should be at the center of medicine when we treat chronic illness. If we don't develop to our potential, it creates an internal conflict, which lowers vitality. This creates a susceptibility which leads to real symptoms causing us to get sick.

So part of treating someone is to perceive where their development has its limitation, and give a medicine that not only treats the physical ailment, but also removes the limitation for healthy emotional and mental development.

Like my mother, who is a teacher, I also like to teach, which I have done for the past twenty years at various colleges and naturopathic schools.

I graduated from Bastyr University in 1987 with a Doctorate of Naturopathic Medicine. In 1989, I went on to complete a further year of study, specializing in homeopathy, and received a diploma (DHANP) from the Homeopathic Association of Naturopathic Physicians.

Works published:

A Case of Hysteria. Simillimum, The Journal of the Homeopathic Academy of Naturopathic Physicians, Winter 1999. Vol, XII, Issue 4.

Trees and Plants That Heal. 1997 Proving of five new remedies.

Winning Strategies of Case Analysis. A short course for RADAR and the Vithoulkas Expert System. Co-authored by George Vithoulkas.

A Case of Paranoid Schizophrenia. Proceedings of the IFH 1994 Professional Case Conference.

The Breakdown State of Baryta Carbonica. Proceedings of the IFH 1993 Professional Case Conference.

Anxiety and Costochrondritis. Simillimum, The Journal of the Homeopathic Academy of Naturopathic Physicians, Spring 1993.

A Case of Chronic Tendinitis. Proceedings of the IFH 1992 Professional Case Conference.

Psuedotsuga Menziesii, Proving With Cured Cases. IFH Professional Case Conference, 1997.

Arbor Medica Volumes I and II. 2007 Publication. Six new tree remedies.

NPLEX Homeopathic Materia Medica Study Guide. Keynotes on Basic Homeopathic Remedies. 2014 Publication

Positive Drug Action. Rebuilding Healthy Gene Expression. 2016 Publication.

If you have some good success with these remedies send me a summary of what happened: drsteveolsen@gmail.com.

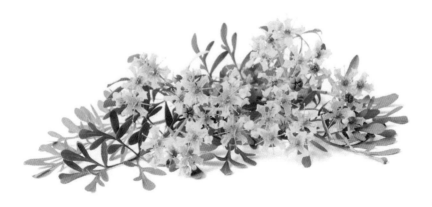

Ruta Graveolens

Index

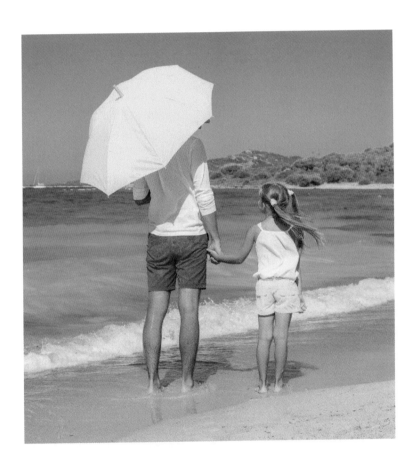

Made in the USA
Charleston, SC
28 October 2016